THE PHARMACIST'S PRESCRIPTION

Your Complete Guide to the Over-the-Counter Remedies that Work Best

F. JAMES GROGAN, Pharm.D.

F. JAMES GROGAN, Pharm.D., received his Doctor of Pharmacy degree from the University of Tennessee and has taught at both the University of New Mexico and Northwestern University. He is presently director of pharmacy ~~~~~~~ ~s at St. Louis State Hospital College of ~~~~~ St. Louis, Missouri.

THE
PHARMACIST'S
PRESCRIPTION

Your Complete Guide to the Over-the-Counter Remedies that Work Best

F. JAMES GROGAN, Pharm.D.

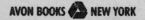
AVON BOOKS ☬ NEW YORK

To Mom and Dad, who taught me to always do my best
To John, who taught me persistence
To Jennifer, Dan, and Claire, who taught me the value of life
And to Donna, who brought it all together.

AVON BOOKS
A division of
The Hearst Corporation
105 Madison Avenue
New York, New York 10016

Copyright © 1987 by F. James Grogan
Published by arrangement with Rawson Associates/Macmillan Publishing Company
Library of Congress Catalog Card Number: 85-82609
ISBN: 0-380-70550-8

First Avon Books Printing: August 1988

AVON TRADEMARK REG. U.S. PAT. OFF. AND IN OTHER COUNTRIES, MARCA REGISTRADA, HECHO EN U.S.A.

Printed in the U.S.A.

K-R 10 9 8 7 6 5 4 3 2 1

Contents

Acknowledgments

Steerage.

Not the ship's compartment that brought my European ancestors to America, but steerage—direction, guidance.

It starts with the family that one is born into—good parents with solid Midwestern values; parents who place a high priority on education and personal excellence; a brother's respect and admiration. Those who lack this background are truly handicapped.

It continues into the school years. Grade school, high school, college. I was fortunate to have good teachers throughout, but especially two consecutive high school English instructors, Fr. Robert Eimer, O.M.I., and Sr. Marie James, S.S.N.D., who pressured and cajoled reluctant high school boys to write intelligible sentences.

The guidance one receives from professional mentors. In my case pharmacists such as Tom Dewein in Belleville, Illinois; Norm Levit in Albuquerque, New Mexico; and Harland Lee in Evanston, Illinois. Each contributed to my professional development in different but equally important ways.

Some are lucky enough to find good people to guide them through unfamiliar territory. Nonfiction writers need the support of expert librarians to help them extract information from intimidating journals, texts, and computer data bases. I could not have completed this book without help from Mary Johnson, Joanne Galanis, Ann Doyle, Mary Sumlin, Terrie Cox, and Vicki Eichhorn at the Missouri

Institute of Psychiatry; and Helen Silverman and Beth Carlin at St. Louis College of Pharmacy.

Advice and encouragement from colleagues and friends: Dean Byron Barnes and professors John Grotpeter and Carol Oliver at St. Louis College of Pharmacy; nurses Mary Ann Stedelin and Virginia Haigler at St. Louis State Hospital; Jerry Warchol, D.M.D., in Belleville, Illinois.

Being virtually steered through the publishing process. Mary Johnson, Eleanor Rawson, and Grace Shaw, who converted my drafts into real English. Michael Larsen and Elizabeth Pomada, who always came through with good advice at desperate moments. Pam Krutsch, who helped with typing, Rick Pfeiffer, Pharm.D., and Steve Ogle, R.Ph., who reviewed the entire manuscript for accuracy. Robert Hutton, M.D., of Dermassociates in Belleville, Illinois, who did the same for the dermatology chapter.

Steerage.

It is continuous. It continues to come from the family that one chooses for one's own. A wife, Donna, who is willing to make the sacrifices necessary to help me achieve my goals.

Steerage.

It comes full circle. Now three young faces, Jennifer, Dan, and Claire, look to me for direction. I pray that I can guide them as well as others have guided me.

My sincerest thanks to each of you.

OTC's—Take with a Large Grain of Salt

> Here, gentlemen, is an ideal drug. It has a
> beautiful color, pleasant odor and delecta-
> ble taste, and although we are convinced
> that it will do the patient no good, we are
> equally certain it will do no harm.
> —William Osler, M.D. (1849–1919),
> speaking of cardamom tincture

Over-the-counter drugs, also known as OTC's or nonprescription drugs, are now, always have been, and always will
be the subject of controversy. Everyone seems to have an
opinion on these agents—and often a vested interest in them.
Consequently there is no shortage of advice spewing forth
upon an unwary and unsuspecting public regarding their use.
Unfortunately, only a small amount of this advice is accurate.

We Americans are a curious combination of advice givers
and seekers. We willingly give and take recommendations
on diets, cars, laundry detergents, and drugs from people
who either have no particular knowledge of the products they
recommend or who have an obvious self-interest in the products they hawk.

It is both expensive and dangerous to give and take suggestions on medication so casually. Every year more than $1
billion are squandered on second-rate OTC drugs, and thousands of people are hospitalized for reactions to drugs they
should not have been taking.

We should be outraged that so many millions are wasted
and that people end up in the hospital from taking what they
believe to be harmless nonprescription drugs. Unfortunately,
the general public has many misconceptions about over-the-

counter drugs, and these misconceptions, or fallacies, are deeply rooted.

Here are just a few common fallacies, with a brief comment on each.

"If these drugs weren't safe they couldn't sell them without a prescription."

No drug is completely safe. Even old, familiar remedies such as aspirin can produce a myriad of side effects and drug interactions. Good old aspirin can kill you if you don't use it properly.

The real difference between prescription and nonprescription drugs is that the latter are *relatively* safe. They still have to be used with caution, and label instructions must be observed.

"If these drugs weren't effective they couldn't be sold."

Who says? It wasn't until 1972 that the United States Food and Drug Administration (FDA) finally got around to checking on the effectiveness of OTC drugs. I'll explain their procedure for reviewing drug efficacy later in this chapter, but let it suffice for now to say that the FDA has had less than heroic success in removing ineffective or marginally effective drugs from the market.

"I can learn all I need to know about an over-the-counter preparation from television commercials."

Oh come on now! Have you ever heard an advertiser say that his product is only second best? With more than 300,000 OTC products out there, choosing the one product that is ideal for your ailment can get pretty hairy. At times like this it can be very helpful to seek a professional opinion—and I don't mean asking the store clerk for a recommendation.

"If OTC drugs were any good they would be limited to prescription status."

It's true that some OTC agents are practically worthless and cause needless side effects, but there are also thousands that effectively and efficiently relieve symptoms of minor discomforts, illnesses, or injuries.

"Old-time products were much more effective than the stuff they put on the market now."

I'm sorry, but the opposite is true. The only active ingredient in many of the "old-time" products was alcohol. Some of the ingredients in those old preparations—beechwood creosote, white pine oil, turpentine, bloodroot, mandrake—would be downright laughable if they were not so toxic.

Unfortunately, you don't have to go back to the good old days to find ridiculous combinations of worthless ingredients. Read the list of ingredients on the packages of the new "herbal" cough drops if you want to have a good laugh at the absurd combination of useless constituents in common use today.

The use of nonprescription drugs is deeply rooted in the tradition of self-care. Since the beginning of history humans have tried to medicate themselves with whatever agents were available. The Department of Commerce estimates that as many as 75 percent of all current illnesses and injuries are self-treated, mostly with OTC drugs.

Some health professionals denigrate the value of OTC medications, but it's clear that our present health care system could not operate effectively without the ready availability of these products. There is no way that our present supply of physicians could efficiently diagnose and treat the threefold increase in patients that would result if nonprescription drugs were not available.

In reality, nonprescription drug use will increase dramatically over the next five years. The Proprietary Association (the trade organization of manufacturers of nonprescription drugs) estimates that OTC sales could increase by almost 85 percent in that time.

At least three factors are responsible for this potential increase: (1) the reclassification of some prescription drugs to OTC status, (2) the increased sophistication of the average consumer, and (3) the economic imperative of avoiding unnecessary physician visits.

In recent years we have seen several frequently used drugs shifted from prescription status to OTC availability. Some of the better known products in this category include hydrocortisone, Tinactin, Drixoral, Afrin, Actifed, and Benadryl. In addition, some OTC antihistamines and decongestants are now available in strengths that used to be limited by law to prescription use. The ready availability of these products allows patients to self-medicate mild to moderately severe conditions that previously could be treated only by a physician.

There can be no doubt about the second factor contributing to the increased use of OTC drugs. Today's consumers are better informed and more interested in all facets of health care than consumers of previous years. The plethora of books and television and radio programs devoted to diets, medications, exercise, and general medical information provides ample testimony to confirm this fact.

Today's consumers correctly insist that the health care system exists to serve their needs. As an integral part of the system, consumers claim the freedom to choose whether they are to be treated by a health care professional or whether they will self-treat their ailments with OTC medications or other treatments. Obviously, consumers may make mistakes in the management of their physical problems, but that is their right and their risk.

The third factor, economics, is probably the most important of the three. Peter Godfrey, former chairman of the Proprietary Association, tells us, ''of every hundred dollars of national income, just under ten is spent for health care. Of that ten dollars, however, less than thirty cents are spent for nonprescription medicines. Yet these products are used to medicate the great majority of personal health problems.''

Thus 75 percent of illnesses in the United States are treated with only 3 percent of the total health care dollar. The fact that self-medication is cost-effective cannot be disputed. Escalating health costs inevitably spur a search for more cost-effective health care, and self-treatment will unquestionably be relied upon to fill much of the bill. Self-medication is a familiar, convenient, and inexpensive method of dealing with mild conditions that are uncomfortable and interfere with daily living.

There's just one problem.

Drugs are like the stereotypical marriage. You love your spouse dearly and want to live with him or her in peace and harmony for the rest of your days. But when you return from your honeymoon you learn that you now have in-laws.

Drugs are not innocuous. It is unrealistic to expect that you gain only the beneficial effects of medication without any risk of side effects. You don't get only what you ask for.

All drugs are chemicals, and the purpose of these chemicals is to alter the function of your body, hopefully for the better. Although OTC drugs are designed by their makers—and required by federal regulation—to be both safe and effective for the treatment of mild ailments, they always have the potential for harm.

Many people fail to recognize that some nonprescription drugs are as strong as the medications your doctor prescribes. This is particularly true for antacids, laxatives, and medications for coughs, colds, allergies, and motion sickness. In some instances, OTC's may be identical to prescription drugs.

Consequently, consumers need a source of factual and unbiased information to help them sort out the good products from the poor ones, to advise them on the proper uses of nonprescription remedies, and to warn them of the risks of potentially hazardous medications. These are the objectives of this book.

My overall purpose here is to provide you with general answers to questions you may have about nonprescription drugs, as well as to provide suggestions for their proper use. This should in no way be construed to mean that this book replaces your medical advisers, because it cannot. Physical conditions and the medications used to treat them are far too complex to be simply and succinctly categorized in a single book.

In the chapters that follow I indicate the products and ingredients I believe are superior to others and explain why I believe them to be so. As the end result, you should have enough information to make an informed choice among commercial products and, even more important, you should more readily be able to determine when to seek professional assistance.

Advertising and Self-Medication

In my opinion, the greatest deterrent to proper self-medication is television advertising.

Much advertising ignores the spirit if not the letter of the law. Most misleading advertisements cannot be forced off the airwaves, because what they say is true—it just is not the full truth. Not only are OTC's hawked as aggressively as underarm deodorants and trash bags, but the resulting overuse of drugs poses a health hazard to consumers.

Products that are heavily promoted are often inferior. If this stuff is so darned good, why does it have to be pushed so hard? In later chapters I will recommend products that you may never have heard of. The reason is that some manufacturers still believe in the philosophy of chocolatier Milton Hershey, who felt that a good product sells itself—you don't need to advertise it.

It would be bad enough if the only deleterious effect of misleading advertising were the pilfering from consumers' pockets. Far greater harm is done to the health of those who use potentially dangerous drugs. *All drugs cause side effects* and a number of these can be lethal for some individuals.

My advice to you is to be skeptical. If a medication sounds too good to be true, it probably is. Advertising should never be confused with education. Never let an ad convince you that you have a condition or disease that you did not previously recognize. Don't be fooled by a commercial of the kind that used to say it is time for a sleeping pill if you cannot get to sleep in fifteen minutes. Such advertising is pure nonsense.

In recent years one company has advertised its plain aspirin product by saying that no combination product is more effective than Brand X aspirin and that buffering is unnecessary. And yet at the same time this same company was advertising a combination product, telling consumers they deserved "extra strength" and "gentle buffers." This is one way of working both sides of the street. A manufacturer can hedge its bets by trying to get you to believe one claim or the other. Obviously, if one of these ads is true, the other must be false. The whole idea is to get you to walk away with one of the company's products.

To top it all, Food and Drug Administration surveys indicate that more than one out of every three adults believe that advertisements about drugs and health aids must be true or the advertiser would not be permitted to make those claims!

The Generic Option

We may never be able to rely on advertisers' speaking truthfully in our lifetime, but we can buy safe and effective drugs without paying for the advertising overhead. The way to combat Madison Avenue prescribing is to buy generic products whenever possible and practical.

Consider that of the more than 300,000 individual nonprescription drugs on the American market, there are only 700 different active ingredients! If you can learn to read labels, you can reduce your dependence on television advertisers.

You are probably already aware that a generic drug is chemically identical to the corresponding nationally advertised brand(s). Generic drugs are less expensive because their makers don't advertise them, nor do the producers take the risk of inventing new products. They just copy older, better known drugs once their patents expire. You benefit from the reduced price.

Ten years ago there was a great deal of concern about generic drugs because some of the generic manufacturers were less than ethical. This situation has vastly improved since the FDA began strict enforcement of its Good Manufacturing Practices guidelines. These regulations have standardized the production of drugs, and the result has been a general improvement in quality throughout the pharmaceutical industry.

To illustrate how you can save money by buying generic products, I visited a pharmacy in my hometown and compared the retail prices of the "name brand" drugs listed in the first column with the generic products sitting next to them on the shelf. The figures speak for themselves.

Name Brand	Quantity	Price	Generic
Peri-Colace	100	$13.60	$2.70
Tylenol	100	4.68	1.92

Dulcolax	100	10.08	1.68
Dramamine	100	22.35	1.26
Drixoral	100	20.85	6.93
Percogesic	100	8.39	4.03
Cortaid cream	1 oz.	4.58	1.33

The pharmacist uses the same percentage markup on all of the products listed above. The difference in prices, therefore, reflects the difference in his actual acquisition costs. Now, tell me where you think your money is going.

The Government's Role in Advertising

What is our government doing about drug advertising abuses? On the surface it would seem that our federal agencies have fumbled the ball.

Two government bureaus have been assigned responsibility for monitoring nonprescription drugs and their advertising. The Food and Drug Administration (FDA) is responsible for assuring that drugs are both safe and effective for their intended purposes. The Federal Trade Commission (FTC) monitors advertising to prevent deceptive or misleading claims.

The FDA's responsibilities are massive when you consider that the agency is in charge of monitoring those 300,000 OTC products as well as several thousand prescription drugs. There is no way any single government bureau, even one the size of the FDA, can effectively fill a job that large.

As a partial solution to this situation, in 1972 the FDA established sixty-nine OTC advisory panels. These panels, composed of practicing and academic pharmacists, physicians, and pharmacologists, reviewed data on OTC products and submitted reports to the FDA. They were responsible for reviewing the ingredients in OTC products to determine whether they could be considered both effective and safe enough for self-treatment. They were also responsible for reviewing advertising claims and for recommending appropriate labeling. (It is the labeling that informs you of a product's active ingredients, its potential uses, and appropriate dosage and warns you about potential side effects and consequences of misuse.)

To give just one example of the recommendations that resulted, the report of the panel on cold remedies recommended that language such as *cold medicine, cold formula,* and *for the relief of colds* be removed from package labels and advertisements, since some purchasers might infer that products so labeled or advertised were a cure when they were not.

The panels were dissolved in late 1984. You may wonder why it took them twelve years to investigate products and to report their findings. There were two primary reasons for the delay and the first is easy enough to understand. These panels of health care experts had to deal with none other than the United States government, and any project that involves the government invariably encounters inordinate delays.

The second reason has to do with the potential impact of the panels' findings. Once a panel submitted its final report, the manufacturers of the "approved" products would be permitted to begin hawking their products as "FDA-approved" or "Found to be safe and effective by a national panel of experts" or "endorsed by the FDA." The panelists needed to be absolutely sure of their findings, or they might find themselves spending a considerable amount of time in court explaining why they found competing products to be dangerous or ineffective.

Although there are shortcomings in the final reports of some of the panels, taken together they have already had a beneficial impact on the nonprescription drug industry. In addition to requiring the reformulation of some products, the panels also recommended that thirty-seven separate drugs or drug dosages that were previously restricted to prescription status be made available over the counter. The panels felt that the public was sophisticated enough to use these drugs safely without strict medical supervision.

The FDA has not acted on all of these recommended status changes, but they have released products such as Benylin Cough Syrup, Benadryl, Sudafed SA, and hydrocortisone ointment.

The flip side of the bureaucratic coin is the Federal Trade Commission. The FTC is assigned the gargantuan task of monitoring the authenticity of drug advertising in all media, not just radio and television. Can you imagine sifting through all the piles of trash cranked out by hundreds of advertising agencies? Can you imagine watching hours of television commercials in an effort to weed out deceptive statements?

Neither can the FTC.

With the coming of the Age of Consumerism we have also seen the advent of the Age of Galloping Gullibility. Studies indicate that consumers may be more easily ripped off now than ever before. Why? Because we think we are being protected more adequately than we really are.

The truth is that the FTC has neither the funding nor the manpower to monitor adequately all the nonsense that appears in interstate advertising. And whenever the bureau tries to take action against an advertiser, a vicious power struggle ensues.

The FTC has the regulatory jurisdiction to require that advertisers submit evidence of tests, studies, or other data to substantiate specific advertising claims. The FTC also has the authority to issue ''cease and desist'' orders when it feels that scientific data do not support these claims. However, each advertiser has the right to fight any FTC ruling in court. The result is often a lengthy proceeding that ties up the commission's resources for years.

The FTC simply does not have the manpower or fiscal reserves necessary to regulate properly all the exaggerated claims we see and hear for OTC drugs. In the meantime, the wise consumer must be skeptical of advertising claims that sound too good to be true.

Where Can You Turn for Advice on OTC's?

This book represents a kind of OTC primer designed to stimulate your interest in proper self-medication and alert you to some potential problems. However, this book has the same limitation as every other health-related book.

That limitation is you.

No two persons react to a drug in exactly the same way, nor do they present exactly the same symptoms of illness. The information in this or any other book is necessarily general in nature and may not apply to your specific case or ailment.

It is prudent for you to consult a medical adviser for professional advice when you have a distressing malady. Sometimes, however, a doctor may not be readily accessible—or you may feel that the complaint is too trivial to concern a physician. For those who fall into this latter category, professional advice on self-care is only as far away as the nearest drugstore.

The pharmacist is generally recognized as the most accessible member of the health care system. How many times have you walked into a medical office or hospital without an appointment and been able to talk immediately with a doctor, nurse, physical therapist, social worker, or dietitian?

In addition to being accessible, the pharmacist is the only health care provider whose entire professional education centers around drug products and drug therapy. He or she has more contact with over-the-counter drugs and has more opportunity to assess patients' responses to these drugs than any other health professional.

Besides recommending specific products, the pharmacist is in a position to perform several important services for you. The first is to inform you about product labeling; another has to do with your individuality.

Many people ignore product labels. Too few consumers fully read label statements or warnings concerning proper dosages or potential side effects. The pharmacist can provide you a valuable service by indicating pertinent information and answering your questions. People heed cautions and warnings better when they understand their purposes. Besides indicating common side effects, your pharmacist can also provide supplemental information such as proper application, appropriate storage conditions, and duration of therapy.

The next vital service the pharmacist can provide is to evaluate your specific case to determine the appropriate treatment or dose. For example, three groups of patients—the very young, the very old, and pregnant women—are often identified as being at relatively high risk of adverse drug reactions. People in these categories should *always* seek professional advice before self-medicating.

Perhaps the best service a pharmacist can provide is to refer you to your doctor when that is the most appropriate course of action. Pharmacists do this frequently when patients present them with symptoms of illness that can't be adequately or safely self-treated.

The Proper Use of Medicine

The New York Pharmaceutical Society found that 85 percent of 10,000 people surveyed either didn't follow the advice written on the labels of medicine containers or didn't comprehend the significance of the instructions. Is it any wonder that people don't respond to medicines or that they unnecessarily suffer side effects from them?

I have fifteen rules to help you get maximum benefit from your medication while minimizing the risk of side effects.

Rule 1. When consulting your pharmacist or doctor, be sure to mention any medical problems you have, as well as all medicines, recreational drugs, or alcohol you are now using or have used in the past few weeks.

Some patients intentionally conceal their use of OTC remedies; others do not regard them as "real drugs." These medications have the potential to interact with prescription drugs or to worsen some physical conditions. You should always report your use of them to your medical adviser.

Drugs you have been taking recently may have caused or aggravated your present problem. Some drugs may have a prolonged action, even if you stopped taking them several weeks ago. Reporting your use of them can greatly facilitate proper diagnosis and treatment.

Rule 2. Before undergoing any surgery, dental procedure, or emergency treatment, be sure to tell your doctor, dentist, or other medical professional who is treating you what medication you are taking.

Rule 3. Remember that *all* drug products contain more than just the active ingredient. Many medications contain salt, sugar, alcohol, or dyes that can cause problems for susceptible individuals. If you have poorly controlled diabetes, are on a salt-restricted diet, or are sensitive to chemical additives that may be in some products, check with your pharmacist or doctor before taking any drug for the first time.

Rule 4. If you are pregnant, or plan to become so, check with your pharmacist and doctor before taking *any* new drug, and review all of your current medications with a health professional in order to prevent harm to your baby. (We will discuss this in more detail in chapter 6.)

Rule 5. If you are breast-feeding a baby, review your medications with your pharmacist, doctor, or nurse.

Rule 6. Follow the directions on your medication container's label unless otherwise instructed by your pharmacist or doctor. Before you leave the pharmacy, be sure you understand all of the instructions and warnings.

Do not take more than the recommended dose. I have one patient who, until I explained the risk, routinely took five Extra Strength Tylenol tablets per dose for her aches and pains. The total *daily* recommended dose of Extra Strength Tylenol is only six tablets. She's lucky she didn't seriously damage her liver.

Rule 7. Always insist on child-resistant containers for all of your medications, and keep your drugs out of reach of children. (I'll explain the reasons for this in chapter 11.)

Rule 8. Store all of your medicines away from bright lights and away from heat and humidity. Because it is easily accessible to children, the bathroom medicine cabinet is the worst place in the house for medicines. A locked closet or cabinet in another room is much better. Follow the storage instructions on the product label.

Rule 9. Don't remove labels from OTC medicine containers. These labels are important because they identify the drug, give proper dosing instructions, list the symptoms the medicine relieves, and list the active ingredients.

Unlabeled or mislabeled containers are an invitation to errors. I'll never forget the day my brother took a swig of shampoo that had been poured into a soda bottle.

Rule 10. Never take medicine in the dark. My uncle once mistook Ben-Gay for his hemorrhoid ointment! He has learned to turn on the light before taking anything.

Rule 11. If you think you have taken an overdose or if a child has taken a medication by accident, call your pharmacist, doctor, hospital emergency room, or poison control center *immediately.*

Rule 12. If your medication is not working or if you notice unusual or unexpected effects from the drug, it may be because of

- Not following the correct dosage schedule
- Interactions with foods, beverages, or other drugs
- Trying to self-medicate when your problem needs a doctor's attention
- Complications that demand further medical attention

Rule 13. If you are more than sixty years of age, ask about any special dosage instructions. Changes in the way your liver or kidneys function may make it necessary to reduce doses.

Rule 14. Ask your pharmacist if he or she keeps patient records. Most reliable pharmacies maintain patient profiles for your protection, and they like to keep track of all of your medications, including OTC's. Also inform the pharmacist of any allergies, medical conditions, or unusual reactions to drugs.

Rule 15. Don't feel embarrassed about asking your medical advisers about your medicines or your medical condition. It is always better to ask and be safe than to suffer a drug reaction in ignorance.

The Toxicity and Side Effects of OTC's

Many patients, and even some physicians, don't consider OTC drugs to have significant toxicity when compared to prescription medications. That impression may have some validity when drugs are used properly, but no medicine is as safe or effective as it should be without responsible and informed consumer use. The thousands of hospital admissions that result every year from reactions to nonprescription drugs contradict any naïve belief in the absolute safety of these products.

Because many products sold over the counter aren't labeled with proper restrictions or warnings about the products' uses, we see far too many hospital admissions resulting from drug toxicity. Researchers have estimated that *20 percent of all drug-related admissions to hospital medical services are the result of reactions to OTC drugs.*

Nonprescription drugs can be just as lethal as prescription medications. Most reactions to OTC's occur for one or more of the following reasons:

* Many of these agents contain more than one ingredient. This causes the patient to be exposed to multiple drugs, some of which may not be necessary. It also increases the likelihood of injurious drug interactions.
* Instructions on the product label may not be clear. You should *always* read all of the information on labels, but sometimes the language used may be stilted or confusing. Not all labels tell you when to stop taking medication or when to consult your doctor.
* Because future sales of the product may depend on whether you feel an immediate effect, the maker may add unnecessary ingredients to boost the product's effect. This is one reason some products contain both aspirin and caffeine. The caffeine has no great effect on pain, but its stimulative effect may make you feel a bit more energetic.
* Some products contain ingredients that can mask the symptoms of an underlying illness. A good example are products that contain phenazopyridine, a urinary anesthetic. If a patient uses one of these products to relieve the pain of a urinary tract infection without taking the proper antibiotics, it is quite possible that he or she (the patient in such cases is almost always a woman) could develop a serious, even life-threatening kidney infection.

Side effects of drug products come not only from the "active" ingredients in them but also from the "inert" substances that are added as preservatives, stabilizers, fillers, or flavors.

Alcohol is used in more than 500 proprietary products and may be found in concentrations up to 68 percent (136 proof). NyQuil, for example, contains 25 percent alcohol (50 proof), while terpin hydrate elixir for coughs is 43 percent alcohol (86 proof). This amount of alcohol can potentially interact with the prescription drug Diabinese, used for diabetes; the antimicrobial drug Flagyl; and Antabuse, the drug used to dissuade alcoholics from drinking.

Alcohol can increase the sedation one experiences with

sleeping pills, tranquilizers, antidepressants, and drugs used for the treatment of epilepsy. It also increases insulin requirements in patients who have poorly controlled diabetes, and it can aggravate stomach ulcers.

Sugar is frequently added to liquid products to improve their taste. Products that are called "syrups" contain sugar, sometimes in concentrations as high as 45 percent. Cough drops and throat lozenges may be 70 percent sugar.

These quantities of sugar may cause problems for some people with poorly controlled diabetes. They are also associated with increases in tooth decay and other dental diseases. My dentist routinely recommends sugar-free medicines to his patients.

To top it all, some products contain *both* alcohol and sugar.

The Risk of Drug-Tampering

One more problem that comes from time to time is the enigma of tampering. We know the results of past adulterations of Extra Strength Tylenol, Anacin-3, and some eye drops. No container is ever completely tamperproof, but you can reduce risk substantially by following the advice of the Food and Drug Administration. The FDA recommends that you watch for the following signs of possible tampering with medicines on store shelves:

- Broken seals
- Open, torn, or damaged boxes
- Loose, torn, or missing wrappers
- Discolored products
- Products with unusual odors

Don't use any internal medicine if the special seal is broken or missing. Remember, however, that some products such as ointments and lotions are exempt from safety seal regulations.

How to Use This Book

This book does not replace your medical advisers, because it cannot. Nor is it intended to replace specific instructions, directions, or warnings that have been given to you by your pharmacist or doctor.

The information in this book is selective; it cannot include all known precautions, contraindications, effects, side effects, or interactions of the drugs discussed. Moreover, it is not practical to list all 300,000 OTC drugs currently on the market.

The most important section of each chapter is the segment dealing with the best-known and most often used drugs available and the recommendations for their use (or non-use) in treatment. I have tried to explain succinctly the effects of drugs marketed for the treatment of common disorders, and I have based my recommendations on reports from the FDA advisory panels, the publications of the American Pharmaceutical Association, data from well-respected pharmaceutical and medical textbooks and journals, and my own experiences and observations, garnered from years of working with patients in hospitals, clinics, and community pharmacies. My recommendations generally reflect the mainstream of current pharmaceutical and medical thinking, but I would be greatly surprised if some pharmacists and physicians did not agree with some of my statements and opinions.

I have tried to make maximal use of lists to help you find information quickly. These lists include information on side effects, drug interactions, recommendations for treatment, and specific products that I do or do not recommend.

Many products that fall into the "Not Recommended for Self-Medication" category may be both safe and effective for some individuals with specific medical problems. "Not Recommended for Self-Medication" is *not* a synonym for *bad* or *dangerous* or *deadly*. In fact, your personal pharmacist or physician may have good reasons for suggesting one of these products for your specific problem.

Nonetheless, the products listed in the "Not Recommended" tables are not recommended by me for one or more of the following reasons, for each of which I've provided a letter key for summary coding purposes: (A) One or more ingredients have been reported to be ineffective or only slightly effective for the product's intended purpose; (B) a more effective product is available; (C) the product advertising or description is likely to heighten consumer expectation beyond actual effectiveness; (D) the product has the potential to cause side effects in the average consumer that are more serious than those generally associated with OTC drugs; (E) the product has the potential to cause serious side effects in persons with specific diseases or disorders; (F) another product is available that is capable of producing the same or nearly the same therapeutic effect without the same risk of side effects; (G) persistent use of the product may cause physical dependency that alters an otherwise normal body function; (H) the product's formulation may reduce the effectiveness of one of its ingredients; (I) this is a multiple-ingredient product that may have no therapeutic advantage over simpler or single-ingredient products; (J) one or more of the product's ingredients may be useful for only a short period during the total duration of the illness; (K) the product cannot easily be administered at a dosage level within generally recommended boundaries of optimal therapeutic effect; (L) this is a condition-specific product that is appropriate for use only after a health professional has helped the patient establish a diagnosis.

The purpose of the product tables and their letter designations is to give you guidance in selecting products for your ailments. In many cases, you may find that a "Not Recommended" product satisfies your needs. Sometimes the difference between a "Recommended" and a "Not Recommended" product is subtle, and other health professionals may have no reservations about recommending one of my "Not Recommended" products.

In addition, these tables are titled "Not Recommended for Self-Medication." In other words, I don't recommend that you select them for *self-use* without consulting with a health professional. You should feel free to discuss any health problem with your pharmacist or doctor, especially if you have questions about specific products and their suitability for your disorder or condition.

In the drug product tables I have tried to list products that are nationally advertised or are readily available throughout the country. There are many examples of generic brands or store brands of drugs that are every bit as good as those I have listed. I would suggest that you either check the generic ingredients of the recommended products or ask your pharmacist for less expensive generics when they are available.

You also need to be aware that manufacturers of OTC drugs frequently reformulate their products without changing a product's name or even indicating a new formulation. Some products may either improve or decline in quality as a result of reformulation. It is important that you read labels carefully and know what you are getting before you buy anything off the shelf.

2

Coughs, Colds, and Hay Fever

The only way to treat a cold is
with contempt.
—William Osler, M.D.
(1849–1919)

The common cold is not called "common" for nothing. Colds afflict more people each year than any other illness. In fact, they occur with such frequency that it is impossible to keep accurate statistics on their annual incidence.

This year American consumers will spend approximately $1.3 *billion* on cough and cold remedies alone. They will lose more time from school and work because of the common cold than from all other diseases combined. More than 250,000 work days will be lost this year due to colds, and approximately 15 percent of the American population will be laid low by them every week this winter.

While some people develop colds in the summer (actually, many of these are allergies, not colds), the vast majority of colds occur in a period beginning in November and ending in April. Within this time frame there are three distinct peak periods for developing a cold. The first is autumn, shortly after schools open. The second is midwinter, when, according to U.S. Public Health Service estimates, half of the population develops at least one cold. The third peak is seen in the spring, just when people prematurely think they are safe.

Children between the ages of one and five years are most susceptible to colds. A child in this age group averages six to twelve episodes each year, and is also more prone than those in other age groups to suffer the complications of a cold, such as middle ear infections *(otitis media)*, pneumonia, and bronchitis. Individuals twenty-five to thirty years old average about six respiratory infections a year, while older adults average two or three.

Factors that favor the development of colds include poor nutrition, fatigue, and emotional disturbances. The presence of these risk factors also increases both the severity of colds and the likelihood of complications such as ear infections, pneumonia, and sinus infections.

Many myths have arisen over the years in an effort to explain the origins of colds. Some say that bathing or showering in the morning reduces your body temperature and causes a cold. Many insist that going outside with wet hair will surely produce a cold and that just being exposed to the north wind increases your susceptibility to colds. And all of us have been told at one time or other that sitting in a draft is the best way to catch a cold. If all these were true, then, presumably, washing your hair while standing in a draft from a north wind would guarantee your getting pneumonia.

While cold air and cold weather are stress factors and may reduce some of the body's natural immunity to colds, the fact remains that *you must be exposed to a pathogenic (illness-creating) virus before you can contract a cold.* Unfortunately, more than 120 different viral strains have been associated with the common cold, and it only takes one of these little gremlins to make you miserable.

The Life Cycle of a Cold

The incubation period—the time between exposure to the virus and the onset of symptoms—is a relatively short one to four days. A cold is most contagious one to two days *prior* to the development of symptoms; it is then that you are most likely to pass on the infection to friends and family.

The earliest symptoms usually are vague feelings of fatigue, muscle aches, and a feeling of "feverishness," even though there is little or no fever.

These symptoms are followed by complaints that are more recognizable as those of a cold. At this stage of the illness you develop congestion in the nose that is first manifested as dryness, followed by a running nose with uncomfortably large amounts of either watery or viscous mucus discharge. This stream of material is the hallmark of the common cold. Although it usually is clear at first, it may later become thicker in consistency and may also be colored yellow or green or some shade in between. The discoloration indicates that red and white blood cells are present and that a bacterial infection may have occurred after the initial viral insult.

Symptoms of a Cold

- General fatigue, or the "blahs"
- Feeling feverish, with little or no actual fever
- Mild stiffness or pain in the back, chest, or legs
- Nasal congestion, with dryness of nasal passages
- Runny nose, with large amounts of clear or colored mucus
- Sinus pressure due to spread of infection into the sinuses
- Spasms of sneezing
- Husky voice or laryngitis
- Sore, scratchy throat

When a nasal discharge, irritation, and congestion combine, sneezing and general misery begin. Irritation in the nasal passages triggers the sneeze reflex. Although it may be hard to believe, sneezing does have a purpose. A good sneeze helps to clear the nose and nasal cavity of foreign material and debris. Unfortunately, the sneeze reflex goes out of kilter during a cold, and sneezing fits may be prolonged, unproductive, and infuriating.

As the infection travels down the respiratory tract, other anatomical structures may be affected. If the larynx, or voice box, is involved, a person may develop a deep, husky voice or even laryngitis.

More commonly, the virus infects the throat, causing scratchy pain, with additional discomfort when swallowing or speaking. This condition is aggravated by the presence of the irritating mucus discharge from the sinuses. (Sore throat and coughs associated with colds will be discussed in more detail later in this chapter.)

Viruses not only spread down the respiratory tract but also can march northward. When they do, they attack the sinus cavities and cause inflammation with increased mucus production. This inflammation commonly shuts off the drainage tract for mucus and causes pressure to develop in the sinus cavities. The pressure brings about a feeling of fullness in the head, resulting in headaches. For many people this sinus congestion is the most uncomfortable symptom of the illness. (Allergy is another cause of sinus congestion and will be discussed later.)

In most healthy people the course of illness in a cold is only five to seven days. A small percentage of patients, however, develop complications that require more specific treatment by a physician.

The most common complications are secondary bacterial infections. The sites for these infections are the ears and tonsils in children, and the sinuses and lungs in adults. Bacterial complications in children are usually accompanied by intense pain in the ears or throat, but symptoms of bacterial infection may be more subtle in adults.

An adult should consult a physician if his or her cold symptoms last for more than ten days, if the nasal mucus changes from a clear fluid to a yellow or green color, or if a cough develops that produces large amounts of colored sputum or phlegm. Any of these signs could indicate that the cold virus has allowed a bacterial infection to complicate things.

Treating a Cold

There is no shortage of advice for cold sufferers. I have heard my nine-year-old lecture her friends on how to handle a cold, and she isn't even sure what a cold is. You may have heard some of the following folk remedies for colds:

- Feed a cold (never mind that you can't taste anything).
- Starve a fever. (What if you have a cold with a fever?)

- Sip whiskey or brandy. (This is more anesthetic than anything else.)
- Eat lemons or drink lemon juice. (This is a form of medical sadism.)
- Eat nutmeg. (Raw nutmeg is a hallucinogen.)
- Get plenty of bed rest. (This one has merit.)
- Soak in a hot bath. (Why not at least be comfortable?)
- Soak in a cold bath. (Which is it, hot or cold?)
- Sip hot honey.
- Eat heated wheat germ.
- Take vitamin C. (We'll deal with this later.)
- Use a back plaster. (Be careful. These can burn and blister your skin!)
- Jog. (This would seem to be the opposite of bed rest!)

Since the potential market, and therefore profit, for cold remedies is so large, an astonishing amount of quackery is involved in formulating and promoting cold remedies. The pirates of the airwaves glibly cajole vulnerable sufferers to purchase quantities of virtually useless and potentially dangerous elixirs and unguents. According to one highly respected medical textbook, "The numerous compounded remedies, including those with vitamins, bioflavinoids, antihistamines, decongestants, and tranquilizers are developed for sales profit in a large market of uninformed and uncritical people."

Think about that the next time you see a commercial for a product that treats "all" the symptoms of a cold.

In treating a cold you need to have a reasonable objective for therapy. Since total cure is out, you need to have an idea of which symptoms can be relieved, which drug will do this, how much of the drug is necessary to produce that effect without undue side effects, and finally, which commercial product(s) achieve(s) these objectives.

The treatment of a simple cold should be simple. This may sound like heresy if you watch a lot of television, but it's true. It may surprise you to know that you don't need to treat all twelve symptoms of a cold, as one commercial exhorts, because you probably won't have all twelve. Even if you do, you won't have them all at the same time. Why should you expose yourself to all of the side effects and expense of superfluous ingredients?

Beware of any ingredient that doesn't make sense to you. If it doesn't seem to belong in the product, it probably doesn't. Some cold products contain laxatives, antacids, quinine, or papaverine. Quinine is useful for treating malaria and leg cramps; papaverine dilates blood vessels in people with poor circulation. None of this has anything to do with a cold. If you aren't sure whether an ingredient belongs in a specific product, ask your pharmacist. Don't take a product just because it's cleverly advertised on television or because a friend says it works for him or her.

The five basic types of drugs commonly used in cold remedies are:

1. Antihistamines, which have little effect on colds
2. Decongestants, which can relieve symptoms for varying lengths of time
3. Anticholinergics, which have no place in the treatment of colds
4. Analgesic antipyretics, which can help relieve cold-related aches and fever
5. Vitamin C, for which great claims are made but little evidence of effectiveness exists

Antihistamines—Little Effect on Colds

Antihistamines are excellent for hay fever and other allergic disorders. They act by blocking the action of the histamine released in the body during an allergy attack. Unfortunately, there is no histamine released during a cold, so antihistamines usually have little effect on colds. A little detail like that doesn't seem to get in the way of the drug companies. Some products even contain two antihistamines, so you can have twice as many side effects without benefit of therapeutic response. (We will discuss use of antihistamines in treating allergies in the section on hay fever, later in this chapter.)

Decongestants—The Best Relief for Some Symptoms

Decongestants are the drugs of choice for treating colds, but the effectiveness of any decongestant varies with the individual and the severity of the illness. Decongestants usually provide some relief from symptoms, although the user may at times be disappointed with the results. It's important to remember that these drugs can *relieve* only some of the symptoms of a cold: *they can't cure it.* It may also be a bit disconcerting to know that your doctor has nothing stronger in his or her prescription armamentarium than the products you can buy over the counter. The effective agent in virtually any prescription decongestant also is available in the same dose in an OTC formulation.

Decongestants may be used in a variety of forms. While I generally prefer the oral forms (liquids, tablets, capsules), many health professionals recommend topical administration (nose drops, sprays, inhalers). We'll cover the relative advantages and disadvantages of these products shortly.

The decongestants are synthetic replicas of the natural substance epinephrine, also known as adrenaline. To oversimplify somewhat, epinephrine and the decongestants stimulate the smooth muscle in blood vessels. This forces the blood vessels to constrict and causes the swollen nasal membranes to shrink. The shrinkage reduces the amount of fluid in the nasal tissues. The end result of these falling dominoes is a normalization of the nasal passages and improved breathing.

The desired effect of decongestants is constriction of the blood vessels in the nose and nasal passages. Unfortunately, these drugs are not selective for the nasal passages and can cause constriction of blood vessels as well as other adrenaline-like effects in other parts of the body. One of the most dangerous possible side effects of these drugs is stimulation of the heart and blood vessels. All decongestants have the potential to constrict arteries not only in the nose, but also in the skin, muscles, and vital organs throughout the body. While this could increase blood pressure, the effects on people with normal blood pressure aren't significant. However, *people who already have high blood pressure should not use decongestants without the advice and knowledge of their physicians.*

As mentioned, decongestants are also capable of stimulating the heart muscle. This can increase the heart rate and increase the amount of blood the heart has to pump. The faster heart rate may not be noticeable to people with a normally functioning heart, but it can be dangerous for those with high blood pressure. They should not use these drugs without checking with a physician.

These drugs also can stimulate the nervous system and cause some of the symptoms we normally associate with anxiety. Susceptible people can have muscle tremors, itching, a feeling of nervousness, and even sweating.

There is a natural tendency to take a decongestant at bedtime to help you breathe during the night and rest more comfortably. Some people end up with less sleep when they do this than if they had done nothing. Why? Because for some people, these drugs are stimulants. One way to avoid staring at the ceiling all night is to take a first "test" dose sometime during the day. If you don't have any problems with stimulation or feelings of anxiety or tension during the day, you probably won't have a problem with a bedtime dose. Never take your first dose of a decongestant at bedtime. You may be sorry.

The box on page 28 summarizes some of the side effects that can occur with decongestants. If you have any questions or concerns about any of them, you should discuss them with your pharmacist or doctor.

Caution! Decongestants and Preexisting Conditions

Decongestants can aggravate preexisting medical conditions. Some of these are listed below. You would be wise not to use any product that contains a decongestant if you think you may have any of these conditions. Remember that a cold is a self-limited illness; it eventually will go away on its own, and it seldom causes severe complications. It's a sad state when people inflict serious, permanent harm on themselves by using drugs when the condition they are trying to treat is only temporary.

Do not use decongestants without your doctor's approval if you have:

• High blood pressure
• Any heart disease
• Angina pectoris

- Coronary artery disease
- Diabetes mellitus (sugar diabetes)
- Overactive thyroid gland
- Previous serious side effects from amphetamine, diet capsules, antiasthma medications, or other decongestants

---

Possible Side Effects of Decongestants

Frequent (seldom require a doctor's care):
Difficulty getting to sleep
Nervousness
Restlessness

Less frequent (seldom require a doctor's care):

Dizziness	Nausea or vomiting
Headache	Shakes or tremors
Increased heartbeat	Sweating

Rare (may be serious; call your doctor immediately):

Difficulty breathing	Seeing things that are not there
Feeling of pressure on the chest	Seizures, convulsions, or fits
Irregular heartbeat	
Pain in the chest	Unusually slow heartbeat

Drugs That Can Interact with Decongestants

Three groups of prescription and nonprescription drugs can adversely interact with decongestants. Since you already know that decongestants can increase blood pressure, it is only logical that they can reduce, or even cancel, the effects of drugs used to treat hypertension.

Do not use decongestants with any of the following drugs unless you consult your pharmacist or doctor first:

- Any drug for high blood pressure

Inderal	Esidrix	Hygroton
Lopressor	Reserpine	Capoten
Minipress	Ismelin	Many others

Aldomet   Catapres
Hydrodiuril   Apresoline

• Antidepressants
Nardil   Tofranil   Asendin
Marplan   Norpramin   Ludiomil
Parnate   Pamelor   Desyrel
Elavil   Aventyl   Many others
Endep   Vivactil

• Bronchodilators for lung diseases
Primatene   Brethine   Proventil
  Mist   Bricanyl   Many others
Alupent   Tedral

Decongestants also have the ability to decrease some of
the effects of antidepressants, making it harder to treat
some forms of depression. In addition, a dangerous interaction exists between decongestants and three rarely used
antidepressants: Parnate, Nardil, and Marplan. People who
take one of these drugs with a decongestant run the risk
of developing a dramatic and potentially fatal increase in
blood pressure.

The interaction with bronchodilator drugs used to treat
asthma, emphysema, bronchitis, and other respiratory
problems is usually not serious. The actions of the bronchodilator drugs listed above are somewhat similar to the
decongestants, and the combination of these drugs can lead
to a greater incidence of side effects.

Oral versus Topical Decongestants

OTC decongestants are available in the oral (taken by
mouth) and topical (applied directly in the nose) forms.
The oral forms (tablets, capsules, liquids) have to travel
from the stomach and intestinal tract through the whole
body before they can act on the inflamed membranes in
the nose. Obviously, they can affect any tissue or organ
they reach anywhere in the body. They also can cause side
effects in any of these areas.

Topical decongestants. The topical forms (nose drops, sprays, and inhalers) are placed directly in the nose and produce their effects right at the place they are applied. Their main advantages are that they act faster than tablets or capsules and concentrate their effects on the nose rather than scattering through the whole body.

A Comparison of Oral and Topical Decongestants

Topical
Advantages:
  Less absorption into the blood
  Fewer systemic side effects
  Fast onset of action
  More intense effect
Disadvantages
  Rebound congestion
  Rhinitis medicamentosa (see page 32)
  Possibility of systemic side effects
  Possibility of contamination of dropper or nozzle
  Tendency to overuse
  Nasal burning

Oral
Advantages:
  Availability of sustained-release forms
  No rebound congestion
  No *rhinitis medicamentosa*
  Not affected by mucus barrier
  Affects mucous membranes of the whole respiratory tract
Disadvantages:
  Higher incidence of systemic side effects (e.g., abnormal heart rhythm, nervousness, insomnia)
  Slower onset of action
  Less intense action

Many people, including pharmacists and physicians, prefer nose drops to capsules because the drops exert a more intense effect. Because the drug is applied directly to the place it is most needed, there is less drug circulating through the body and less risk of side effects and drug interactions.

Notice that I said "less" risk of bad effects, not "no" risk. It is still possible that nose drops and sprays can cause these effects, because the nose is an excellent site for drug absorption. Any cocaine snorter knows that. Any drug you take nasally always is absorbed through the membranes of the nose, and some small portion also trickles down the throat and is swallowed. Therefore, even topical decongestants can produce side effects on the heart, blood vessels, and other organs, although the side effects usually are not as common or severe as with decongestant tablets or capsules.

Nose drops and sprays relieve stuffy noses faster and better than tablets or capsules can, but this is a mixed blessing. Most people have never been told that this nasal relief often is followed by a condition called "rebound congestion," a form of drug withdrawal in which the nose gets extra-congested when the effects of the drug wear off.

Most people have never heard of this problem and think that the added congestion is just part of their colds. Guess what they do then? Right! They shoot up with more drops or spray, and the rebound congestion comes a little earlier and a little earlier with each dose of decongestant.

This creates a cascade effect. The user shoots up initially because of congestion. The medication gives some temporary relief but causes even more congestion on the rebound when the effect wears off. Our poor cold-sufferer begins to use the drops more frequently, trying to ward off not only the initial congestion but also the drug-induced problem. Pretty soon the user is snorting and spraying far past the time when the original problem should have abated.

This situation is much more common than you may think. Some folks end up almost addicted to their nose drops. I know several people who buy their decongestant drops by the pint!

But that isn't all the bad news. The long-term overuse of nose drops can lead to a more serious condition known as *rhinitis medicamentosa*. This is a condition of rebound congestion complicated by the destruction and complete loss of the microscopic hairs that protect the nasal membranes from dirt and bacteria. The longer this situation lasts the more difficult treatment becomes.

How long does it take for rebound congestion to occur? Most medical textbooks say that it takes about five days of continuous use for the rebound to start, but my experience has been that these symptoms may be seen in as little as two days. That is why I generally recommend decongestants by mouth over nose drops and sprays. I have never heard of a case of rebound congestion from decongestant tablets.

If you have rebound congestion, how do you get rid of it? Unless you have damaged your nasal passages, all you have to do is to stop using the drops. But this is no easy matter. People who try to kick the nose drop habit experience congestion worse than their original cold symptoms. Most people will begin to experience some relief from the congestion in a couple of days, but it takes several more days for the symptoms to disappear completely. Those who have damaged their airways may require an expensive cortisone-type nasal spray to restore normal function to the affected areas.

Special hazards exist in using topical decongestants in infants and small children. Decongestants are capable of causing all of the side effects I mentioned earlier, but they may be more severe than you normally would expect. Kids usually fight and squirm when you try to give them nose drops. Consequently, they often end up getting more medication than they should. In addition to that, a child's nose is different from an adult's; the child usually absorbs more drug through the nose and into the blood than the adult does. Once the drug is in the blood it can raise blood pressure, affect the heart, and do all of the other bad things decongestants can do.

A factor that many parents fail to consider is that most of the standard over-the-counter preparations are available only in adult concentrations. The adult products should not be used for children, because of the potential for overdose. If you are using an adult product or any other medication for children, be sure to read the directions on the label. Some nose drops, such as Neo-Synephrine, are available in special concentrations for children.

A surprising number of people don't know how to take nose drops or sprays properly. The box that follows summarizes the correct way to give or take these products. If you need additional help or information, do not hesitate to talk to your pharmacist or doctor.

The Right Way to Use Nose Drops

1. Blow your nose *gently*.
2. Tilt your head back as far as it will go. This is easier to do if you are sitting in a chair or lying over the edge of a bed.
3. Place the proper number of drops in each nostril, and keep your head tilted back so the medication can spread throughout the nose.
4. Sit up and blow your nose *gently*.
5. Rinse the dropper with hot water and dry with a clean tissue or cloth.
6. Do not use the same container or dropper for more than one person or you may spread the infection to others. Nose drops do not contain antibiotics to prevent contamination.

The Right Way to Use Nasal Sprays

1. Blow your nose *gently*.
2. Keep your head upright and spray the medication into the nose.
3. Wait a few minutes and then blow your nose *gently*.
4. Rinse the top of the container with water and dry with a clean tissue or cloth. Be careful not to get water in the container.
5. Do not use the same container for more than one person or you may spread the infection to others. Nasal sprays do not contain antibiotics to prevent contamination.

The most commonly used topical decongestants are ephedrine, phenylephrine, naphazoline, oxymetazoline, xylometazoline, levodesoxyephedrine, and propylhexedrine. Not exactly names that trip off the tongue, are they? In any event, a summary of the properties of each of these is listed in the table below.

Nonprescription Topical Decongestants

Generic name: **Phenylephrine**
Common brand name(s):
  Alconephrine
  Neo-Synephrine
  NTZ
  Sinarest
Peak effects: 30 minutes
Duration of activity: 30 minutes to 4 hours
Comments: Prolonged exposure to heat and light causes deterioration.

Do not use if the solution contains sediment or has a brown tinge.

Use the weakest effective strength to minimize the severity of rebound congestion.

Among the most effective topical decongestants.

Generic name: **Naphazoline**
Common brand name(s): Privine
Peak effects: 30 minutes
Duration of activity: 2 to 6 hours
Comments: May cause sedation rather than stimulation when absorbed into the blood.

Produces rebound congestion 4 to 6 hours after application.

Not recommended for children under 6.

Generic name: **Oxymetazoline**
Common brand name(s):
  Afrin
  Duration

Neo-Synephrine 12 Hour
Sinex-L.A.
Peak effects: 5 to 6 hours
Duration of activity: 8 to 10 hours
Comments: Patients frequently overlook the long duration
of action and use too frequently.
Overuse leads to rebound congestion and *rhinitis med-
icamentosa.*

Generic name: **Xylometazoline**
Common brand name(s):
Neo-Synephrine II
Sinutab
Peak effects: 5 to 6 hours
Duration of activity: 8 to 10 hours
Comments: Patients frequently overlook the long duration
of action and use too frequently.
Overuse leads to rebound congestion and *rhinitis med-
icamentosa.*

Generic name: **Propylhexedrine**
Common brand name(s): Benzedrex
Peak effects: 15 to 30 minutes
Duration of activity: 2 hours
Comments: This drug vaporizes easily and is used in in-
halers.
Active ingredient can be lost if the cap is not properly
replaced.
Since the effects wear off quickly, there is great po-
tential for overuse and rebound congestion.

Generic name: **Levodesoxyephedrine**
Common brand name(s): Vicks Inhaler
Peak effects: 15 to 30 minutes
Duration of activity: 2 hours
Comments: This drug vaporizes easily and is used in in-
halers.

Active ingredient can be lost if the cap is not properly replaced.

Since the effects wear off quickly, there is great potential for overuse and rebound congestion.

Generic name: **Ephedrine**
Common brand name(s): Vatronol
Peak effects: 1 hour after administration
Duration of activity: 4 to 6 hours
Comments: Less effective than other decongestants.
More side effects than other decongestants.
Deteriorates in direct sunlight. Protect from light and heat.
Not recommended for children under 6.

Levodesoxyephedrine and propylhexedrine vaporize easily and are suitable for inhalers, such as Vicks Inhaler and Benzedrex. Since their effects last only two hours or so, there is a tendency to use them too frequently. Even though inhalers don't look like drugs, they certainly are. These drugs are capable of causing all the side effects described for other decongestants.

Oral decongestants. The oral forms of decongestants (tablets and capsules) have several advantages over the drops and sprays. I normally recommend oral decongestants for people who don't have any medical conditions that preclude their use. The most important advantage of the oral products is the lack of rebound congestion and *rhinitis medicamentosa*.

A few other advantages are unique to the tablets and capsules. The length of time the oral agents remain active in your body is shorter than some of the long-acting drops, but the tablets and capsules can be manufactured in sustained-release forms. These allow the drug to dissolve more slowly in the stomach and intestines. The slower dissolution results in a longer duration of activity, up to twelve hours after a single dose. This provides you with the convenience of only twice-a-day dosing.

When you use nose drops the beneficial effects of the

medication are limited to the areas that come into direct contact with the drug. Oral agents can produce their effects on *all* the mucous membranes lining the nose, nasal cavity, and the sinuses. This more generalized effect allows mucus drainage by relieving the inflammation that is present in the sinuses. Many people with sinus headache find relief this way.

In a sense, the oral decongestants work from the inside out. They are absorbed from the stomach and small intestine and are transported in the blood to all parts of the body, including the nose. Nose drops are placed directly in the nose and must work their way through all the mucus and viral debris in order to go to work. Some people who have large amounts of thick nasal secretions may respond better to oral decongestants than to nose drops.

Many people also experience a burning sensation from nose drops. This is caused by an intense constriction of the blood vessels in the nose and indicates that the blood supply to the nasal membranes is being drastically reduced. Oral decongestants don't cause as intense an effect as the drops, and burning isn't a problem.

A Comparison of Oral Decongestants

Generic name: **Pseudoephedrine**
Common brand name(s):
  Afrinol
  Sudafed
  Sudafed SA
Peak effects: 30 to 60 minutes
Duration of activity: 4 to 6 hours (12 hours for sustained-release products)
Comments: Individuals over 50 years old may be more sensitive to side effects.
  Causes relatively little stimulation and sleep disturbance.
  May have the lowest incidence of side effects among the oral decongestants.

Commonly used as an ingredient in prescription-only products.

Use only for children over 7 years of age unless advised otherwise by your pharmacist or doctor.

Generic name: **Phenylpropanolamine**
Common brand name(s): Propadrine
Peak effects: 30 to 60 minutes
Duration of activity: Up to 3 hours (longer with sustained-release products)
Comments: High incidence of side effects.

Has an appetite suppressant effect.

Has considerable stimulant properties.

A common ingredient in ''kiddie dope'' (see page 273).

Individuals over 50 years old may be more sensitive to side effects.

Not recommended for children under 2 years.

Generic name: **Phenylephrine**
Comments: Rapidly destroyed in the stomach and intestinal tract.

Very little of the drug gets absorbed into the blood.

Least effective of the oral agents.

Not recommended as an oral decongestant.

Anticholinergics—Do Not Use for Colds

The anticholinergic drugs in cold products are isolated from the leaves of the belladonna plant. Avoid any product whose ingredients include atropine, hyoscyamine, scopolamine, and ground up belladonna itself. These drugs have no direct effect on any of the symptoms of a cold—they are included in some cold products because one of their side effects is the drying of nasal secretions. This is intended to decrease nasal drainage and relieve the drippy feeling that you experience in the early days of a cold. Unfortunately, the small doses commonly found in nonprescription products haven't been shown to produce this effect reliably.

The anticholinergics are also associated with a long list of side effects in addition to their drying effect on the nose. These side effects include dry mouth, blurred vision, dilated pupils, constipation, retention of urine, heartburn, heart palpitations, increased or decreased heart rate, headache, flushing of the skin, skin rashes, nervousness, drowsiness, generalized weakness, dizziness, insomnia, fever, restlessness—and nasal congestion.

I once had to send a middle-aged man to the hospital emergency room because he had not been able to urinate in the twenty-four hours since he took a dose of one of these products for a cold. The company that makes the drug has since changed the product's ingredients and removed the belladonna, but some of the generics still contain belladonna. I recommend that no one take any cold product that contains any of the anticholinergics mentioned above.

Anticholinergic drugs have no place in the treatment of colds. They have the potential to cause a great deal of harm and offer very little prospect for doing good. In addition, most products that contain anticholinergics also contain antihistamines. Not only do antihistamines have little value in treating a cold, but they also have anticholinergic-like side effects. Don't let yourself get caught in this double whammy.

Analgesic Antipyretics—Pain and Fever Reducers

Analgesic antipyretics are drugs that relieve both pain (analgesic) and fever (antipyretic). The two most commonly used drugs of this type are aspirin and acetaminophen (Tylenol, Datril, and many other brands). Their actions, interactions, side effects, and more will be discussed in detail in chapter 3. At this point we will only look at their use in colds.

Pain symptoms, especially headache, muscle soreness, and stiffness, are common during colds. Low-grade fevers also occur frequently. Both symptoms can be treated adequately with aspirin or acetaminophen alone.

Many manufacturers include either aspirin or acetaminophen in their products and then advertise that these products treat "all the symptoms of a cold." In reality, the discomfort or fever you experience with a cold normally lasts only a day or two, making it unnecessary to continue taking the extra drugs for the entire duration of the cold.

Don't waste your money on cold products that contain aspirin or acetaminophen. It's more economical and safer just to take aspirin or acetaminophen when you feel you need them and then stop taking them when they are no longer needed.

We'll review the side effects of these drugs in chapter 3, but I should mention here that aspirin has a unique effect on the viruses that cause colds. Researchers have found that aspirin somehow helps to spread your infection to the other folks around you. As far as I know, acetaminophen doesn't do this.

Vitamin C—No Clear Proof of Effectiveness

Linus Pauling says that you should take 1 to 5 grams of vitamin C every day to prevent colds and then take *15 grams per day* to treat a cold. Although Dr. Pauling is the recipient of two Nobel Prizes, neither is for vitamin therapy. (One is for chemistry and the other is the Peace Prize.)

There is considerable talk and intense feeling about the use of vitamin C for colds, but there is little reliable scientific data to indicate that it has a significant effect on colds. Even if we give Dr. Pauling the benefit of the doubt for now and assume that there is some role for vitamin C in cold prevention, the effects of taking this drug, or any other drug, still need to be carefully considered.

Since colds are fairly innocuous, any drug used to prevent them should be both safe and effective. Vitamin C proponents are fond of saying that the vitamin has no side effects and any excess is simply eliminated in the urine. The facts don't bear this out.

High doses of vitamin C commonly cause diarrhea and affect the urinary system. Research indicates that high doses of vitamin C increase the chance of developing kidney stones and may also affect the elimination of other drugs. That means it may interact with some drugs either to increase or decrease their effects. For example, vitamin C may interact with the anticoagulant Coumadin to decrease Coumadin's effects, with the result of placing the patient at risk of having a heart attack, stroke, or blood clot.

Vitamin C also interferes with some tests for diabetes and may cause a diabetic to use the wrong dose of insulin.

There is some evidence that doses in excess of 3 grams of vitamin C daily may decrease fertility in women. It appears that women taking high doses of vitamin C have more difficulty becoming pregnant and are more likely to miscarry once pregnancy occurs. However, vitamin C is not reliable enough to be used as a contraceptive.

Other Cold Remedies

A comforting, effective nondrug treatment for colds is room humidification. Humidifiers increase the moisture content in the air, and this moisture keeps the mucus in the nose and sinuses from drying out. When mucus loses some of its moisture content it becomes thicker and harder to remove when you blow your nose.

Besides the discomfort of not being able to blow this stuff out, there is some evidence that excessive drying of nasal passages may make you more susceptible to complicating bacterial infections. As we've already observed, the antihistamines or anticholinergics found in most cold tablets and capsules also cause nasal drying.

How much room moisture is enough? It is generally thought that 40 to 50 percent room humidity is necessary for normal comfort, but 60 to 80 percent is better for people with colds and other respiratory problems. If you overshoot the 80 percent range, however, water condensation on walls and windows becomes a problem. If the room humidity becomes too high, the air grows oppressive and breathing becomes more difficult.

The two basic types of humidifiers are the old hot steam vaporizers and the newer cool mist humidifiers. The steam vaporizers offer no particular advantage and have the disadvantages of potential electric shock and fire hazards. The cool mist units are safer in households with small children.

While it is the water itself that produces the mucus thinning, several companies market additives for steam vaporizers. As far as I have been able to determine, these additives make the room smell "medicinal" but do little else. It has not been established that these products provide better therapeutic benefit than inhaling plain water mist.

Chest rubs like Vicks Vaporub and Mentholatum Ointment are similar to the vaporizer additives. They are odorants that have mainly psychological benefit.

℧

The Pharmacist's Prescription for a Cold

General Information

Time is the only cure for a cold. Medications may help to relieve some of the discomforts of a cold, but they do not abate them completely.

Medications can cause side effects and further complicate a cold. Stop using them if you experience significant side effects, such as headache, sweating, or irregular heartbeat.

Antibiotics do not help a cold. They are only useful for treating secondary bacterial infections. Do not use leftover antibiotics or a friend's antibiotics without consulting your doctor.

Recommended Treatment

Bed rest is highly recommended. If this is not practical, frequent naps are a suitable alternative. Rest reduces the total amount of sick time, prevents complications, and decreases the chances of passing on the infection to others.

Continue to eat if you have an appetite. Good nutrition is important in treating most illnesses.

Drinking fluids, including fruit juices, is essential. Drink as much as you reasonably can unless your doctor has told you otherwise.

Use a humidifier to help loosen thick mucus. The cool mist units work as well as the steam vaporizers. There is no need to add medication to the water.

Decongestants are the most effective drugs for relieving many of the symptoms of a cold. I recommend the oral decongestants (tablets, capsules) over the topical agents (drops, sprays).

Oral decongestants (in order of preference):
1. Pseudoephedrine
2. Phenylpropanolamine
3. Phenylephrine

Sustained-release products may be more convenient, and in some cases less expensive than an equivalent dose of regular tablets.

Topical decongestants (in order of preference):
1. Phenylephrine
2. Naphazoline
3. Oxymetazoline
4. Xylometazoline
5. Propylhexedrine
6. Levodesoxyephedrine
7. Ephedrine

Aspirin and acetaminophen are very useful in treating the mild muscle aches and fever that can occur with a cold.

A scratchy throat or a tickle in the back of the throat often can respond as well to hard candy or honey as to expensive throat lozenges or cough drops.

See the Doctor if . . .

- Your cold lasts longer than a week.
- You develop a fever higher than 101°.
- You develop a sore throat that persists beyond two days.
- Your nasal or throat mucus becomes yellow or green.
- You develop an unusually stiff neck.
- You develop an unusually severe headache or pain above the teeth, on the sides of the nose, or around one or both eyes. This may be an indication of a sinus infection.
- You develop an earache.

Products Recommended for a Cold
Oral products (products taken by mouth)

Afrinol	Novafed
Neo-Synephrine Day	Sudafed
Relief	Sudafed SA

Or the generic equivalent of any of the above

Topical products (products applied to the nose)

Afrin	Neo-Synephrine II
Afrin Pediatric	Neo-Synephrine 12 Hour
Alconephrin	NTZ
Allerest	Privine
Coricidin	Sinarest
Dristan Long Lasting	Sinex-L.A.
Nasal Mist	Sinutab
Duration	St. Joseph
Neo-Synephrine	Super Anahist

Or the generic equivalent of any of the above

Products Not Recommended for Self-Medication of Colds

Oral Products (products taken by mouth)

Actifed (A,F,I)
Alka-Seltzer Plus (A,F,I,J)
Allerest (A,F,I)
Allerest Headache Strength (A,F,I,J)
Aspirin Free Dristan (A,F,I,J)
Bayer's Children's Cold Tablets (J)
Benadryl (A,F)
BQ Tablets (A,F,I,J)
Chlor-Trimeton (A,F)
Chlor-Trimeton Decongestant (A,F,I)
Congespirin (J)
Contac (A,F,I)
Contac Severe Cold Formula (A,F,I,J)
Coricidin (A,F,J)
Coricidin D (A,F,I,J)
Coryban D (A,F,I,J)
CoTylenol (A,F,I,J)
Dimetane Decongestant (A,F,I)
Dimetapp Extentabs (A,F,I)
Dristan (A,F,I)
Drixoral (A,F,I)
Head and Chest (I,J)
Headway (A,F,I,J)
Novahistine Cold Tablets (A,F,I)
Novahistine Elixir (A,F,I)
NyQuil (A,F,I,J)
Sinarest (A,F,I,J)

Sinarest Extra Strength (A,F,I,J)
Sine-Aid (J)
Sine-Off (A,F,I,J)
Sine-Off Non-Aspirin Formula (A,F,I,J)
Sinutab (A,F,I,J)
Sinutab Extra Strength (A,F,I,J)
Sinutab II (J)
St. Joseph Cold Tablets for Children (J)
Sudafed Plus (A,F,I)
Super Anahist (J)
Triaminic (A,F,I)
Triaminicin (A,F,I,J)
4-Way Cold Tablets (A,F,I,J)
Or the generic equivalent of any of the above

Topical products (products applied to the nose)
Benzedrex (G)
Dristan (A,I)
Dristan Long Lasting Menthol Nasal Mist (I)
Dristan Menthol Nasal Mist (A,I)
Duration Mentholated Vapor Spray (I)
Neo-Synephrine Mentholated (I)
Neo-Synephrine 12 Hour Vapor Nasal Spray (I)
Sine-Off Once-A-Day (I)
Sinex (I)
Vatronol (I)
Vicks Inhaler (G)
Or the generic equivalent of any of the above

Miscellaneous products
VapoRub (A,J)
VapoSteam (A,J)
Or the generic equivalent of any of the above

The products listed in the "Not Recommended" tables are not recommended by me for one or more of the following reasons: (A) One or more ingredients have been reported to be ineffective or only slightly effective for the product's intended purpose; (B) a more effective product is available; (C) the product advertising or description is likely to heighten consumer expectation beyond actual effectiveness; (D) the product has the potential to cause side effects in the average consumer that are more serious than those generally associated with OTC drugs; (E) the product has the potential to cause serious side effects in persons with specific diseases or disorders; (F) another product is available that is capable of producing the same or nearly the same therapeutic effect without the same risk of side effects; (G) persistent use of the product may cause physical dependency that alters an otherwise normal body function; (H) the product's formulation may reduce the effectiveness of one of its ingredients; (I) this is a multiple-ingredient product that may have no therapeutic advantage over simpler or single-ingredient products; (J) one or more of the product's ingredients may be useful for only a short period during the total duration of the illness; (K) the product cannot easily be administered at a dosage level within generally recommended boundaries of optimal therapeutic effect; (L) this is a condition-specific product that is appropriate for use only after a health professional has helped the patient establish a diagnosis.

Coughs

You have probably seen one of those television commercials in which the announcer tries to make you believe that a cough is just about the worst debility ever to beset mankind. He usually goes on to hawk the "strongest cough suppressant available without a prescription."

I'll bet you have never heard a commercial sponsor say that coughing is a natural function of the body and serves a purpose. I haven't either, but it's true. Without being able to cough, we would drown in our own respiratory refuse. A cough allows us to get rid of excess mucus and cellular debris from the lower reaches of the lungs. It also allows us to expel the remains of dead viruses and bacteria that have tried to invade our air passages. Some patients are actually *taught* to cough after surgery to clear their lungs of bacteria and mucus.

People who have a serious illness in which the cough reflex is completely suppressed soon develop pneumonia and die. A cough can be lifesaving when a person needs to eliminate a large amount of secretion or sputum.

Coughing isn't a disease and shouldn't be treated as one. A cough is often a symptom of an illness, and control of the underlying problem is the best approach to the treatment of an overactive cough.

A cough may result from a simple irritation of the throat or some other part of the respiratory system. Coughs may even result from irritation of nerves in other parts of the body, such as the ears. The box opposite lists some causes of persistent cough.

Most coughs originate from an area of the brain cleverly named the "cough center." This center is uncomfortably close to another area that has been identified as being responsible for nausea and vomiting. Prolonged or strenuous coughing can trigger the vomiting center, causing gagging and vomiting.

Coughs are usually described as being congested or dry and as productive or nonproductive. A congested cough is one where fluid or phlegm accumulates and makes rattling sounds in the chest. You can correctly assume a dry cough to be the opposite. Productive refers to the ability to bring up or expectorate that fluid or phlegm. A nonproductive cough is one where the material in the chest does not come up with the cough.

The three basic types of cough are:

1. Congested/productive—a cough associated with chest congestion, with the patient able to cough up some of the mess
2. Congested/nonproductive—a cough associated with chest congestion, but with the patient unable to cough up any of the congestion
3. Dry/nonproductive—when there is no congestion in the chest and nothing comes up with coughing

A dry, nonproductive cough is frequently seen in the recovery phase of viral infections. Some people may develop this type of cough simply as a nervous habit. (Cough medications aren't effective for a nervous cough.)

Reflex coughs are also dry and nonproductive. These are coughs that result from irritation that may or may not originate in the respiratory tract. The coughs may be the result of inhalation of irritants, such as smoke, or from disturbances in the vocal cords, ears, or even the stomach.

It is exasperating to experience a mild cough during the day and then find that it gets worse when you try to go to sleep. This happens because the secretions in the nose and throat tend to pool in the back of the throat when we lie down. The resulting irritation makes us cough more and disturbs our sleep.

Some Causes of Persistent Cough

Infections
  Nasal infections
  Sore throat
  Sinus infections
  Ear infections
  Pneumonia
  Lung abscess
  Bronchitis

Allergies
  Hay fever
  Asthma
  Nasal polyps

Environment
  Cold temperature
  Humidity
  Tobacco smoke
  Dust
  Fumes
  Pneumoconiosis

Developmental
  Tracheo-esophageal fistula
  Cystic fibrosis
  Esophageal diverticulum
  Vocal cord palsy
  Hernia of the diaphragm

Other
  Prolonged use of nose
    drops
  Cancer in the airway
  Irritation of the eardrum
  Aspiration of a foreign body
  Heart failure
  Collapsed lung
  Emphysema

While a cough is a normal response to respiratory irritants, it can be harmful if it gets out of hand. The box lists some of the potential complications of severe coughing episodes.

In addition to treating the underlying illness, there are medications that may be used to treat the cough itself. However, short of paralyzing the respiratory tract, there is no medication that absolutely obliterates every cough.

There is no shortage of products advertised as cough remedies. However, many of them contain ingredients that are either ineffective or counterproductive. Most cough products contain one or more of three types of medica-

Possible Consequences of Severe Coughing

Soft tissue and bones
  Broken ribs

  Rupture of postoperative
    wounds
  Muscle tears

Cardiovascular
  Decreased cardiac blood
    output
  Heart rhythm disturbances
  Fainting

Respiratory tract
  Asthma attacks
  Air in the chest cavity
  Abnormalities of the
    windpipe (trachea)

Other
  Ruptured blood vessels
    (nose, eyes, rectum)
  Loss of sleep
  Fatigue
  Irritability
  Involuntary urination
  Nausea and vomiting
  Hernia

tions. They have been used with varying degrees of success to control the severity of coughing or to maximize the usefulness of the cough reflex. These basic drug groups are:

- Expectorants
- Antitussives
- Demulcents

Cough syrups and cough drops, rather than fitting smoothly into one or other of these groups, are often a combination of two or more types of drugs.

Expectorants—Of Questionable Use

Expectorants assist your body's natural defense system to break up phlegm so that it can be coughed up. (The most commonly used expectorant is guaifenesin.) The use of these drugs has one unfortunate drawback: They have never been proven to work.

While some of the expectorants described here are used in both prescription and nonprescription cough remedies, there is no convincing proof that any of them is superior to large doses of water.

Expectorants supposedly act by drawing water into the lungs and by liquefying the phlegm in the airways. This changes a dry, nonproductive cough to a cough that is more productive and less frequent.

When using an expectorant, it is important to follow the medication with as much water as possible. Cough syrups should *not* "stick in the throat." They have to get to the stomach in order to be absorbed into the bloodstream so they can do their job.

In addition to being used for garden variety coughs, expectorants also may be useful in treating the chronic cough that occurs with cigarette smoking, asthma, chronic bronchitis, or emphysema. Treatment of these conditions should be supervised by a physician.

A Comparison of Expectorants

Generic name: **Guaifenesin**
Common brand names:
  Colrex Expectorant
  2/G
  Robitussin
Side effects: Side effects from guaifenesin are infrequent. They include:
  Diarrhea
  Nausea or vomiting
  Drowsiness
  Stomach pain

Generic name: **Ammonium chloride**
Common brand names: Ammonium chloride usually is not marketed as a single agent. It is an ingredient in the prod-

ucts that follow. Because of its potential side effects and lack of effectiveness, none of these products should be taken without a physician's recommendation.

Baby Cough Syrup
Chlor-Trimeton Expectorant
Chlor-Trimeton Expectorant with Codeine
Efricon
Endotussin-NN
Endotussin-NN Pediatric
Histadyl EC
Kiddies Pediatric
Kophane Syrup
N-N Cough Syrup
Noratuss
Quelidrine
Romilar CF
Triaminicol
Tricodene Sugar Free Syrup

Side effects: Ammonium chloride in high doses can cause severe metabolic side effects in patients with kidney, liver, or chronic heart conditions.

It may change the acidity of the urine and affect the elimination of other drugs from the body.

It can produce nerve disorders in alcoholics or in individuals who drink large amounts of alcohol consistently.

Generic name: **Ipecac syrup**

This is the same drug used to cause vomiting in persons who have swallowed a potential poison (see chapter 11). In smaller doses it is claimed to possess expectorant properties.

Common brand names including this ingredient: The products that contain ipecac as a single ingredient are intended to produce vomiting. They should not be used as a cough remedy. The following products contain small concentrations of ipecac. Since effectiveness of the drug is questionable, none of these products is recommended.

Cerose DM
Cetro-Cerose
Dr. Drake's

Quelidrine
Sorbutuss

Side effects: There is no information on the effects of the amount of ipecac that is absorbed from the intestinal tract in these small doses.

Generic name: **Terpin hydrate**
Common brand names: Usually available by its generic name
Side effects:
Stomach burning
Nausea and vomiting

Comments: Terpin hydrate elixir is also known as GI gin. It has an alcohol content of nearly 45% (90 proof). Terpin hydrate elixir and its codeine-containing counterpart, terpin hydrate with codeine elixir, are frequently abused.

Due to their lack of proven effectiveness and high alcohol content, terpin hydrate and terpin hydrate with codeine elixirs are not recommended.

Other Drugs with Unproven Expectorant Effects

Products containing any one or more of the following ingredients are not recommended for self-medication without the advice and consent of a physician.

Beechwood creosote   Pine tar
Benzoin   Potassium
                            guaiacolsulfonate
Camphor   Sodium citrate
Chloroform   Syrup of squill
Eucalyptus oil   Tolu
Menthol   Turpentine
Peppermint oil   Wild cherry syrup

Water—An Effective Expectorant

You can imagine how beneficial it would be to have a drug that could be used to clear the lungs of the muck left there by colds, pneumonia, bronchitis, asthma, emphysema, tuberculosis, and a host of other respiratory diseases. If we had such an agent, patients with these conditions would probably improve faster and more comfortably.

Fortunately, there is one such agent, but you'll never see it advertised on television. It's plain tap water.

While this may come as a surprise to you, doctors have known about the expectorant properties of water for years. It is one of their best kept secrets.

The action of water in the lungs is really rather simple. When you drink water some of it is drawn to the lungs, where it mixes with the mucus in the bronchi. The mixing of water with the lung contents results in the dilution, or watering down, of the mucus that clogs small airways. This reduces the thickness of the phlegm and makes it easier to cough up.

How much should you drink? The average person needs to drink six to twelve glasses of water a day to achieve this effect. Another way to judge if you are taking in enough fluids is to drink water until your urine loses its normal yellow color and becomes colorless.

When water is used in large quantities as an expectorant, it becomes a medicine and may have side effects. If your doctor has advised you to restrict your fluids, you should check with him or her before using water this way.

Another way to use water as an expectorant is by means of a steam vaporizer or cool mist humidifier, discussed earlier in this chapter.

Antitussives—For Limited Use Only

While on the surface the cough suppressants known as antitussives may seem the ideal drugs for the treatment of any cough, they usually are not.

Antitussives dull the cough reflex and allow phlegm and bacterial and viral particles to stay in the lungs, where they can continue to cause problems. These drugs thwart one of the body's important defenses, and you should use them only when your cough is of the dry, nonproductive kind. In special circumstances they may be used for the other types of coughs—if the coughing spasms are so strenuous that sleep is disturbed or if there is danger that the cough may cause physical harm.

Demulcents—For Minor Throat Irritations

Demulcents are most effective for the tickling sensations in your throat that lead to those irritating little coughs that drive you crazy. Demulcents coat and soothe your throat. They usually are made up of little more than sugar, and hard candy, such as Life Savers, probably works as well as any of the cough drops presently on the market.

Cough Syrups and Cough Drops—A Confusion of Formulations

In too many cases the cough syrups on the market act as demulcents rather than as "cough medicine." Some of these products contain as much as 85 percent sugar and provide up to 15 calories per teaspoonful. Dentists have shown that these sugar-containing drugs cause tooth decay in adults and children.

Cough medicines may also contain a host of other ingredients that contribute little to the treatment of a cough. It's common, for instance, to find cough syrups that contain antihistamines and decongestants so you can treat a whole mess of symptoms with one dose. We discussed some of the problems with this earlier in the chapter, and the same reservations apply here.

Some cough medicines also contain significant amounts of alcohol. In some cases small amounts of alcohol are necessary for the stability of the ingredients. Some other products, however, contain as much as 45 percent (90 proof) alcohol, providing up to 30 calories per teaspoonful.

Besides having no known therapeutic effect on coughs, high alcohol concentrations can cause serious problems for some people. Alcohol can interact with tranquilizers, sleeping medications, antidepressants, anticoagulants or blood thinners, and diabetes medications.

A particularly poor form of treatment is the cough drop or lozenge that contains a cough suppressant with or without other medications. The problem here is that some people pop these things like candy whenever they feel a little tickle in the throat or have a muffled cough. This is no problem with the candy-type cough drops like Luden's, Vicks, or Halls, but one can overmedicate with the antitussive in lozenges like Hold or Spec-T.

The Pharmacist's Prescription for Coughs

General Information

A cough is a natural protective mechanism and should normally *be assisted* rather than obliterated.

Drinking large amounts of water and breathing humidified air make a cough work more efficiently and often decrease the amount of coughing.

Combination products should generally be avoided. Decongestants, antihistamines, and alcohol have no role in the treatment of coughs. They may increase discomfort by causing side effects.

Common sense dictates that smokers should stop smoking, if not permanently, at least until the cough has disappeared.

Recommended Treatment

Treatment depends upon the type of cough:

Congested/nonproductive

Use an expectorant to break up the congestion in the lungs and allow the body to cough up phlegm. Water is the best expectorant, but some doctors and pharmacists feel that guaifenesin may be used in addition to water.

Antitussives (cough suppressants) should only be used if the cough is hyperactive, that is, if it is so severe or frequent that it impairs normal functioning.

Congested/productive

Use an expectorant such as water to bring up mucus material. Antitussives should only be used if the cough is hyperactive.

Dry/nonproductive

Antitussives are often effective when the cause is an irritation in the throat.

Demulcents such as honey, hard candy, or the candy-type cough drops may also be beneficial.

See the Doctor if . . .
- Your cough lasts for more than seven days.
- Your cough is so severe that it causes you to gag, choke, or vomit or if it interrupts your sleep.
- You cough up blood.
- You have any of the complications previously listed.

Products Recommended for a Cough

Expectorants (each contains guaifenesin)
  Colrex Expectorant
  2/G
  Robitussin

Antitussives (each contains dextromethorphan)

Benylin DM	Pinex
Delsym	Romilar Children's
Pertussin 8-Hour Cough	St. Joseph Cough Syrup
Formula	for Children

Or the generic equivalent of any of the above

Products Not Recommended for Self-Medication of Coughs

Bayer Cough Syrup for Children (I,J)	Coricidin (I,J)
Benylin (F)	DayCare Capsules (I,J)
Breacol (I,J)	DayCare Liquid (I,J)
Cheracol (I)	Dimacol (I,J)
Cheracol-D (I)	Dorcol Pediatric Cough Syrup (I,J)
Chlor-Trimeton Expectorant (I,J)	Dristan Cough Formula (I,J)
Chlor-Trimeton Expectorant with Codeine (I,J)	Formula 44 Cough Control Discs (I)
Conar (I,J)	Formula 44 Cough Mixture (I,J)
Conar Expectorant (I,J)	

Formula 44-D (I,J)

2/G-DM (I)

Halls (I,J)

Naldecon CX (I,J)

Naldecon DX (I,J)

Naldecon EX (I,J)

Naldetuss (I,J)

Novahistine Cough
   Formula (I,J)

Novahistine Cough and
   Cold Formula (I,J)

Novahistine DH (I,J)

Novahistine DMX (I,J)

Novahistine Expectorant
   (I,J)

Orthoxicol (I,J)

Pertussin Cough Syrup
   for Children (I)

Quiet-Nite (I,J)

Robitussin AC (I)

Robitussin CF (I,J)

Robitussin DAC (I,J)

Robitussin DM (I)

Robitussin PE (I,J)

Romilar CF (I)

Sudafed Cough Syrup
   (I,J)

Triaminic Expectorant
   (I,J)

Triaminic Expectorant
   with Codeine (I,J)

Triaminicol (I,J)

Trind-DM (I,J)

Tussar-2 (I,J)

Tussar-SF (I,J)

Vicks Cough Syrup (I)

Vicks Cough Silencer
   Lozenges (I)

Viromed Liquid (I,J)

Viromed Tablets (I,J)

The products listed in the "Not Recommended" tables are not recommended by me for one or more of the following reasons: (A) One or more ingredients have been reported to be ineffective or only slightly effective for the product's intended purpose; (B) a more effective product is available; (C) the product advertising or description is likely to heighten consumer expectation beyond actual effectiveness; (D) the product has the potential to cause side effects in the average consumer that are more serious than those generally associated with OTC drugs; (E) the product has the potential to cause serious side effects in persons with specific diseases or disorders; (F) another product is available that is capable of producing the same or nearly the same therapeutic effect without the same risk of side effects; (G) persistent use of the product may cause physical dependency that alters an otherwise normal body function; (H) the product's formulation may reduce the effectiveness of one of its ingredients; (I) this is a multiple-ingredient product that may have no therapeutic advantage over simpler or single-ingredient products; (J) one or more of the product's ingredients may be useful for only a short period during the total duration of the illness; (K) the product cannot easily be administered at a dosage level within generally recommended boundaries of optimal therapeutic effect; (L) this is a condition-specific product that is appropriate for use only after a health professional has helped the patient establish a diagnosis.

Sore Throat

The irritation or discomfort of a sore throat, more properly called pharyngitis, is usually the result of either viral or bacterial infection. In some cases the discomfort may be caused by irritants such as tobacco smoke or air pollution.

Most sore throats are minor nuisances and require no more than candy cough drops. The most common symptoms of a sore throat are soreness and dryness rather than actual pain.

The great majority of sore throats are caused by viruses, so antibiotics are totally ineffective against them. Most infectious disease experts don't even recommend antibiotics for most bacterial sore throats. In fact, the only common type of sore throat that requires antibiotics is strep throat.

While neither you nor your doctor can diagnose a strep throat just by looking at it, there are some symptoms that do suggest that this might be the problem. Strep throat is often associated with a rapid onset of illness and intense pain in the throat. Patients usually feel weak and may run a high fever. They may also have hard, swollen lymph glands on the sides of the neck.

On the other hand, viral sore throats seldom cause high fever, are usually associated with a cold or the flu, and usually come on slowly. Patients with viral infections normally have no difficulty swallowing and complain of a scratchy feeling rather than intense pain.

If you have symptoms that resemble those of a strep throat, see a doctor as soon as possible. Most other cases of sore throat can be treated for symptomatic relief with an over-the-counter drug.

OTC's that are marketed for the treatment of sore throat are only effective for relieving some of the discomfort in the throat. They do not shorten the course of the illness by even one minute. The various types of OTC's include cough drops, throat lozenges, gargles, and tablets and capsules.

Most of the candy-type cough drops (Luden's, Vicks,

Halls, and many others) act as demulcents on the throat. In other words, their soothing properties are due largely to their sugar content. They reduce the discomfort of a sore throat in much the same way sipping tea and honey does.

Some well-designed scientific studies have indicated that a warm saltwater gargle, which costs you less than a quarter for a gallon of solution, is just as effective as gargling with some of the commercial mouthwashes/gargles. The secret is in the preparation of the saltwater.

The solution should be prepared by adding one teaspoonful of salt to a cup of warm water. Too much salt causes burning in the throat, and too little is ineffective. These saltwater gargles have the dual effect of soothing the inflammation in the throat and of cutting through some of the mucus that may be coating and irritating the sensitive throat membranes.

Other commercial gargles and throat lozenges may contain a local anesthetic that is supposed to numb the nerves in the throat. Unfortunately, they also deaden the nerves in the tongue and mouth. Some people have choked on food after using a prescription anesthetic gargle. *Don't try to eat for at least an hour after using an anesthetic gargle.*

Nevertheless, anesthetic gargles can give significant relief from sore throat pain if they are used properly. It does no good just to swish the stuff around in your mouth and then spit it out. In order to get any relief, you must allow the gargle to go part of the way down your throat and then swish it by making a "gargling" sound. An anesthetic can't relieve pain if it doesn't come into contact with the painful area.

The most commonly used anesthetics are phenol and benzocaine. Both are effective but should not be used in either the gargle or lozenge form more than once every four hours. Unfortunately, they are only effective for one to two hours.

Aspirin and acetaminophen (Tylenol, Datril, and many others) are probably more effective in relieving sore throat pain than any of the medications described above. Chapter

3 deals with their use in detail. For now it's sufficient to say that these drugs must be swallowed in order to work.

There is no benefit from gargling aspirin solutions or in letting an aspirin tablet dissolve in your mouth to relieve sore throat pain. When aspirin, an acid, is allowed to come into contact with a sore, inflamed throat, it is likely to cause even more pain and discomfort. The only relief you can expect to get is from the aspirin that is eventually swallowed and is allowed to work like a regular aspirin tablet.

There is no reason that I know of that you cannot use more than one type of sore throat remedy at a time. You can, for instance, take aspirin, gargle with warm saltwater, and suck on hard candy or a medicated throat lozenge if you wish.

♉

The Pharmacist's Prescription for Sore Throats

General Information

Most sore throats are due to viral infections and antibiotics have no effect in their treatment.

Many sore throats caused by bacteria do not require antibiotic therapy.

Your doctor can only be sure if you have a "strep throat" by taking a throat culture.

Hard candy, "medicated" throat lozenges, saltwater gargles, "medicated" gargles, and aspirin or acetaminophen may be used together if you so desire and will not interfere with any antibiotic that your doctor may prescribe.

Recommended Treatment

Rest is very helpful in clearing a sore throat. This includes limiting the use of your voice as much as possible.

Tobacco smoke is irritating to the throat. Stop smoking if you possibly can.

Aspirin and acetaminophen are the most effective treatments for the pain of a sore throat. (See chapter 3 for information on proper doses and possible side effects.)

See the Doctor if . . .
- Your sore throat lasts for more than one week.
- You also have a high fever, chills, or hard, swollen glands on the sides of your neck.
- You have any difficulty breathing.
- You have difficulty swallowing fluids.

Recommended Throat Lozenges

Cepacol Troches
Cepastat
Cherry Chloraseptic
Children's Cepastat
Children's Chloraseptic
Isodettes Super
Menthol Chloraseptic

Mycinettes Sugar Free
Oracin
Semets
Spec-T Sore Throat
   Anesthetic
Vicks Throat Lozenges

Throat Lozenges Not Recommended for Self-Medication

Cepacol (B)
Children's Hold 4 Hour Cough Suppressant (I)
Chloraseptic Cough Control (I)
Hold (I)
Hold 4 Hour Cough Suppressant (I)
Robitussin-DM Cough Calmers (I)
Spec-T Sore Throat/Cough Suppressant (I)
Sucrets (A)
Sucrets Cough Control Formula (I)
Sucrets Cold Decongestant Formula (I)
Thantis (A,I)
Throat Discs (I)

The products listed in the "Not Recommended" tables are not recommended by me for one or more of the following reasons: (A) One or more ingredients have been reported to be ineffective or only slightly effective for the product's intended purpose; (B) a more effective product is available; (C) the product advertising or description is likely to heighten consumer expectation beyond actual effectiveness; (D) the product has the potential to cause side effects in the average consumer that are more serious than those generally associated with OTC drugs; (E) the product has the potential to cause serious side effects in persons with specific diseases or disorders; (F) another product is available that is capable of producing the same or nearly the same therapeutic effect without the same risk of side effects; (G) persistent use of the product may cause physical dependency that alters an otherwise normal body function; (H) the product's formulation may reduce the effectiveness of one of its ingredients; (I) this is a multiple-ingredient product that may have no therapeutic advantage over simpler or single-ingredient products; (J) one or more of product's ingredients may be useful for only a short period during the total duration of the illness; (K) the product cannot easily be administered at a dosage level within generally recommended boundaries of optimal therapeutic effect; (L) this is a condition-specific product that is appropriate for use only after a health professional has helped the patient establish a diagnosis.

Hay Fever

Hay fever, also known as rose fever, is an allergic disorder that occurs most frequently in the summer and fall. Its symptoms coincide with the times of the year when pollen and mold spore counts are at their peak. The most common symptoms are sneezing, a runny or congested nose, and itching and tearing of the eyes.

Sounds a lot like a cold, doesn't it? The basic difference between the two conditions is that a cold is an infection, while hay fever is an allergy. Because the basic cause of illness is different, they require totally different treatments.

The terms *hay fever* and *rose fever* are actually misnomers. Neither hay nor roses commonly cause these problems, and there is seldom any fever present. The disorder is more properly called *allergic rhinitis*, or a runny nose caused by allergies. Other medically correct terms are *pollen allergy* and *pollenosis*. For our purposes we'll continue to call it hay fever.

Hay fever fortunately occurs in only a small percentage of people who are exposed to plant pollens. Not all pollens are capable of causing these allergic reactions and, in general, hay fever attacks are most frequently caused by the pollens released by weeds, grasses, and trees. As a general rule, flowering plants that must be pollinated by bees and other insects don't release their pollen into the air and infrequently cause problems.

The weeds, grasses, and trees that cause hay fever are usually wind-pollinated. In other words, they release their pollen into the air in the hope that the wind will carry it to another plant. A single ragweed plant can release as many as 1 million grains of pollen in a single day. Ragweed pollen has even been found at sea, as much as 400 miles from land! It's impossible to eliminate ragweed pollen by killing all the plants around your home or even in your town. The stuff can come from miles away.

Ragweed is the most common plant allergen in this country, but there are plenty of others around. Some others are sagebrush, redroot pigweed, careless weed, spiny amaranth, tumbleweed, plantain, and goldenrod. No region of the country is spared. If you decide to "send your sinuses to Arizona," you should expect to develop new allergies to plants like sagebrush or tumbleweed.

The next most important group of pollens are those that come from grasses. Frequent offenders include timothy grass, redtop, Bermuda, orchard, and some varieties of bluegrass.

Trees that can cause problems for susceptible folks include walnut, hickory, oak, and pecan, as well as elm, poplar, box elder, and mountain cedar.

The molds that live on decaying vegetation and in damp basements also produce airborne spores that cause the same symptoms as the pollens.

As the pollen and mold spore counts rise, hay fever sufferers usually experience more frequent and more severe attacks. Pollen counts may vary widely depending upon the weather conditions on any particular day. For instance, they drop dramatically after a heavy rain because the rain water "washes" them out of the air. This may be a mixed blessing, however, since moisture usually allows molds to grow even more vigorously and to produce more spores.

Pollens and molds aren't the only respiratory allergens we have to watch for. Susceptible people can also react to house dust, animal danders, feathers, insects, bath powders, sawdust, insecticides, tobacco smoke, hydrocarbons, and practically anything else that flies through the air. There have even been some reports of allergic reactions to minute food particles released into the air by cooking.

If why some people react to these allergens and others do not puzzles you, don't feel bad. The hot-shot scientists haven't figured it out either.

Where the experts have been more successful is in determining the sequence of events that trigger allergic reactions. They tell us that when pollen particles are inhaled they stick to the mucus and hairs in the nasal passages. Enzymes in these protective bodies try to dissolve the foreign particles so the body can get rid of them. Unfortunately, some pollens contain specific allergenic substances that are released when the pollen's coat is dissolved. The presence of these foreign substances triggers the release of chemical defenders that try to destroy them. In most people this is the end of the story, but in allergic individuals, the body overreacts with a full-blown allergic reaction.

As I mentioned earlier, the most common symptoms of hay fever are sneezing, itchy nose, and a watery discharge of mucus from the nose and sinuses. Sudden attacks of sneezing may consist of ten to twenty sneezes in rapid succession. This sneezing is often accompanied by itching, burning, and watery eyes.

Some people may also have a condition known as perennial rhinitis, in which they experience a continuous nasal congestion with postnasal drip. These folks seldom have the sneezing attacks or the profusely watery nose and eyes.

Hay fever isn't a contagious disease. You can't catch it from—or spread it to—anyone else. It isn't necessary to stay away from people during these episodes.

For most people, hay fever doesn't lead to anything more serious. However, about a third of those with this condition may develop asthma at a later point in life. Some are also susceptible to sinus or ear infections if the passageways to these areas are closed during hay fever attacks. It is, therefore, advisable to check with your doctor for proper diagnosis and follow-up of this or any other allergy.

The treatment of hay fever usually consists of a combination of the following:

- Avoiding the substance to which you are allergic
- Undergoing a series of ''allergy shots'' designed to change the way your body reacts to allergens
- Using medications to prevent or minimize the symptoms of the allergy attacks

Some of the ways you can reduce your exposure to allergens include closing the bedroom windows at night, staying away from burning leaves and grass, and staying indoors during the times of the year when pollen and mold counts are at their highest. The filters in air conditioners can be helpful in removing some of the pollen from the air in your home. A special electrostatic filter is even more effective. However, be cautious when changing these filters, because you can react to the materials that they have trapped. It is usually advisable to get someone else to change them for you.

About 70 to 80 percent of allergy sufferers experience some relief from allergy shots. The first step in this form of treatment, however, is to identify the agents that are causing the problems. This is usually done by running a series of skin tests. The components of the allergy shots are then individualized for each patient based on the results of these tests. Each injection is slightly stronger than the one preceding it until the patient can tolerate normal exposures to the offending allergens.

Antihistamines—Relief with Possible Side Effects

The form of treatment that most patients and physicians opt for initially is the use of an over-the-counter antihistamine. Many of these products are highly effective for the control of the symptoms of allergies and happen to be some of the very same drugs listed as "Not Recommended for Self-Medication" in the section on colds.

These anithistamines are often marketed by their manufacturers as "cold and allergy" medicines. In reality, they should simply be called "allergy" medications, because they are much more effective for allergies than they are for colds.

Antihistamines are generally considered to be the drugs of choice for the treatment of hay fever and some other allergic conditions. Many of these products also contain the same decongestants discussed in the section on the common cold. While decongestants don't do much for the hay fever itself, they can be very useful for those who need relief from nasal congestion.

Numerous antihistamines have been developed and introduced to the American market since 1942. Initially, they were thought to cure the common cold, but we now know that they have little beneficial effect on that condition.

Histamine is a naturally occurring chemical in the body. While it normally helps to protect us from outside invaders, this process sometimes fails to work. Inappropriate histamine release can cause itching, sneezing, watery eyes, and skin rashes. Antihistamines work by competing with histamine in the respiratory tract and other areas of the body. They sometimes prevent, but do not reverse, histamine's effects.

While these drugs have helped millions of people over the years, their effects have been disappointing in many ways. In some instances antihistamines don't reach their site of action in the nasal passages in high enough concentrations to have a significant effect. There is also some question about whether the antihistamine drug can get into the same areas that collect histamine. Moreover, histamine is only one of the chemicals involved in allergic reactions, and antihistamines are effective in blocking the effect of histamine alone.

Antihistamines work only by antagonizing chemicals normally present in the body; they have no intrinsic beneficial effects of their own. Antihistamines aren't capable of totally reversing allergic reactions, but they are able to prevent allergic symptoms if given early enough.

As a general rule, antihistamines are quite effective if they are given an hour or so before an anticipated exposure. For instance, if you are allergic to cat dander, you might do well to take a dose of antihistamine just before you visit a cat-loving friend. By the same token, hay fever sufferers experience less discomfort if they take an antihistamine before going for a ride in the country.

Some antihistamines are only effective for a few hours after a dose. Manufacturers have tried to circumvent this problem by developing "specially coated" tablets or "time-release" capsules that attempt to prolong the action of the drug for eight to twelve hours. Unfortunately, not all of these sustained action products actually work for the full amount of time the label promises.

Just as antihistamines are useful in treating a variety of

allergic disorders, they all possess a wide variety of side effects. The most common undesirable side effect is sedation. This is an unpleasant experience for most people in that it impairs their ability to concentrate and also decreases their ability to perform physical tasks. Even if the drug is taken at bedtime, it can cause some degree of drowsiness the next day. Fortunately, most people develop a tolerance for this effect with time and experience little problem after the first few days of treatment.

Antihistamines may cause either drowsiness or a paradoxical stimulation in children. The reasons for this stimulation are poorly understood. This effect often explains why some children's behavior worsens when they take these drugs.

The table that follows lists some of the side effects of antihistamines, potential interactions with other drugs, and some of the medical conditions antihistamines can aggravate. If you are at all concerned about any of these items, be sure to consult your personal pharmacist or physician.

The Hazards of Antihistamines

Side Effects
Frequent (seldom require a doctor's care):
  Drowsiness
  Thickening of mucus secretions
Less frequent (seldom require a doctor's care):
  Blurred vision
  Difficult or painful urination
  Difficulty sleeping
  Dizziness
  Dryness of nose, throat, or mouth
  Fast heartbeat
  Loss of appetite
  Nausea
  Nervousness or unusual activity, especially in children
    or the elderly
  Rashes
  Stomach pain or burning

Sweating

Rare (may be serious; *call a doctor immediately*):
Unexplained sudden onset of sore throat and fever
Unusual bleeding or bruising
Unusual weakness

Drug Interactions
Alcohol
Sedatives
Tranquilizers
Antidepressants
Medications for sleep
Medications for seizures
Narcotic drugs
Prescription pain medications
Other antihistamines

Medical Conditions
Do not take an antihistamine if you have any of the following medical conditions unless you first consult your physician:
Bladder problems
Glaucoma
Heart disease
High blood pressure
Obstruction in the gastrointestinal tract
Obstruction of the bladder or urinary system
Overactive thyroid gland
Prostate problems
Ulcers

Symptoms of Overdose
(Children are more at risk than adults.)
Excitement
Incoordination
Twitching
Convulsions
Flushed Skin
Comas

Decongestants—Sometimes Helpful for Hay Fever

Decongestants don't have any direct effect on the course of allergic reactions, but they can be helpful to some people with hay fever. Those who have nasal congestion and sinus pressure during their bouts of allergic rhinitis often experience great relief with products that combine an antihistamine with a decongestant.

Some effective products are listed below. Some of the products that are not recommended contain more than one antihistamine and/or decongestant. There is no advantage in combining two similar drugs, because one is adequate if the dose is sufficient.

The side effects of decongestants were discussed earlier in this chapter. You can find a listing of them on page 28.

The Pharmacist's Prescription for Hay Fever

General Information

There is no cure for hay fever. The best treatment is decreased exposure to possible allergens.

Medications may help relieve some of the symptoms of allergies but do not reverse them entirely.

Antihistamines frequently cause uncomfortable side effects. You are the only one who can judge whether the side effects are better or worse than the symptoms you are experiencing.

Antibiotics have no value in the treatment of hay fever unless along with it you also develop a respiratory or sinus infection.

Recommended Treatment

Antihistamines are the most effective agents currently available for the treatment of hay fever. Chlorpheniramine and brompheniramine are the least sedating antihistamines available without a prescription.

Decongestants may be effective for those who have nasal or sinus congestion associated with the hay fever. If these conditions are not present, decongestants have no value and have the potential to cause serious side effects.

Analgesics such as aspirin, acetaminophen (Tylenol and

others), or ibuprofen (Advil, Nuprin) may be used for the headaches and aches and pains that may accompany hay fever. I do not recommend a combination antihistamine and analgesic in the same product because you usually do not need to use the analgesic for as long as you need the antihistamine.

See the Doctor if . . .
- You get no relief from over-the-counter drugs.
- Your nasal mucus changes color.
- You develop pain above your teeth, on the sides of your nose, or around your eyes.
- You develop an earache.
- You develop intolerable drowsiness or sedation.

Products Recommended for Hay Fever
Antihistamine-only products
   Chlor-Trimeton
   Pfeiffer Allergy Tablets
     Or the generic equivalent of either of the above

Combination antihistamine-decongestant products

Actifed	Novafed A
Allerest	Novahistine Cold Tablets
Chlor-Trimeton	Novahistine Elixir
Decongestant	Novahistine Fortis
Contac	Novahistine Melet
Demazin	Sudafed Plus
Dimetane Decongestant	Triaminicin Allergy
Dimetapp	Triaminicin Chewables
Dristan Time Capsule	Trind
Drixoral	Tri-Nefrin
Fedahist	

     Or the generic equivalent of any of the above

Products Not Recommended for Self-Medication of Hay Fever

Alka-Seltzer Plus (I)	Congespirin (I)
Allerest Headache	Coricidin (I)
Strength (I)	Coricidin D (I)
Aspirin-Free Dristan (I)	Coryban-D (I)

CoTylenol (I)
Dristan-AF Tablets (I)
Dristan Capsules (I)
Headway (I)
Novahistine Sinus Tablets (I)
Sinarest (I)
Sinarest Extra Strength (I)
Sine-Aid (I)

Sine-Off (I)
Sine-Off Extra Strength (I)
Sine-Off Non-Aspirin Formula (I)
Sinulin (I)
Sinurex (I)
Sinutab (I)
Sinutab Extra Strength (I)
Sinutab II (I)
Triaminicin (I)

The products listed in the "Not Recommended" tables are not recommended by me for one or more of the following reasons: (A) One or more ingredients have been reported to be ineffective or only slightly effective for the product's intended purpose; (B) a more effective product is available; (C) the product advertising or description is likely to heighten consumer expectation beyond actual effectiveness; (D) the product has the potential to cause side effects in the average consumer that are more serious than those generally associated with OTC drugs; (E) the product has the potential to cause serious side effects in persons with specific diseases or disorders; (F) another product is available that is capable of producing the same or nearly the same therapeutic effect without the same risk of side effects; (G) persistent use of the product may cause physical dependency that alters an otherwise normal body function; (H) the product's formulation may reduce the effectiveness of one of its ingredients; (I) this is a multiple-ingredient product that may have no therapeutic advantage over simpler or single-ingredient products; (J) one or more of the product's ingredients may be useful for only a short period during the total duration of the illness; (K) the product cannot easily be administered at a dosage level within generally recommended boundaries of optimal therapeutic effect; (L) this is a condition-specific product that is appropriate for use only after a health professional has helped the patient establish a diagnosis.

3

Dealing with Aches, Pains, and Fever

Humanity has but three great enemies;
fever, famine and war;
of these by far the greatest,
by far the most terrible,
is fever.
—William Osler, M.D. (1849–1919)

This year the American public will spend nearly $2 billion on over-the-counter pain relievers. The stakes are too high for advertisers and manufacturers to sit idly on the sidelines. More money is spent on advertising OTC pain relievers (analgesics) than any other single group of OTC drugs.

Whenever that kind of money is at stake, you can bet that there will be no shortage of hucksters in there grabbing for their share of it. Do any of the following sales pitches sound familiar to you?

- "Acts five times faster than aspirin"
- "Arthritis pain formula"
- "Arthritis strength"
- "Enhanced relief of pain"
- "Fast pain relief"
- "Long-lasting pain relief"
- "Reaches peak action twelve times faster than aspirin"
- "So gentle it can be taken on an empty stomach"
- "Special pain-relieving formula"

The odds are that you have been persuaded by at least one of these advertising claims. You may be interested to know that the FDA advisory committee has judged each of them to be false or misleading.

This panel *does* feel that it is appropriate and accurate for advertisers to claim that their products are effective for the *temporary* relief of occasional minor aches, pains, headache, and for the reduction of fever. The panel calls on the Federal Trade Commission to exercise more control over drug advertisements, particularly those shown on programs that are likely to be seen by large numbers of children.

Causes and Types of Pain

Pain is an important part of the body's natural warning system. Pain usually occurs when some part of the body is either being damaged or is in danger of being injured. *Since pain may be an indication that something is wrong, you should not be too quick to jump in to treat it without also trying to determine its cause.*

While pain is a feeling that is familiar to all of us, most of us do not appreciate the complexity of how we perceive pain or how we relieve it.

The feeling of pain begins with the stimulation of specialized nerve fibers. Nerve endings in the skin, muscles, bones, and internal organs are capable of detecting noxious stimuli. They telegraph their message through specialized nerve fibers in the spinal cord to sensory areas of the brain. The brain is responsible for interpreting these messages and, in return, issuing a feeling of pain.

Headache

Headache is the most common cause of pain, as well as the most frequent reason for using an over-the-counter analgesic drug. Each week 15 percent of the American population experiences a headache.

Most people tend to think of headache as simply a pain in the head. In reality, headaches can be quite complex. The large number of medical specialty journals and specialized headache clinics attests to this fact.

While it is beyond our scope to discuss headaches in

anything approaching that degree of detail, we can describe a few of the more common types.

Some Types of Headache

Brain tumor	Migraine	Tension
Cluster	Psychogenic	Traumatic
Histamine	Sinus	Vascular
Meningeal irritation	Temporal arteritis	

Traumatic Headache

This most serious type of headache should not be self-medicated. Any headache that occurs after a head injury and is accompanied by impaired consciousness or alertness, abnormal responses of the eyes to light, confusion, or by bleeding from the ears, mouth, or eyes requires immediate medical attention. Trying to treat this type of headache yourself not only delays proper medical treatment, but may also complicate proper diagnosis and treatment of the basic problem. If you have a head injury, contact a doctor as soon as possible.

Tension Headache

Tension headache is the most common type of headache and is familiar to most of us. Since the pain is caused by spasms of the muscles surrounding the skull, it would be more proper to call this a "muscle contraction headache."

The pain of a tension headache is usually located either in the forehead or the neck. Symptoms include a feeling of tightness or pressure at the base of the head. The muscles of your neck and even your back can be involved.

This headache can be caused by eye or muscle strain. Vacationers who are unaccustomed to driving long distances at night and those who try to read in poor light often develop tension headache. Tension headache is also the bane of front-seat theater patrons.

Vascular Headache

Unlike tension headache, vascular headache occurs when the blood vessels inside the skull dilate and put pressure directly on the brain. Vascular headache can be caused by a wide variety of disorders. For instance, vascular headache can result from fever, blood poisoning, caffeine withdrawal, and vasodilating drugs such as nitroglycerin and niacin. Migraine and cluster headaches are types of vascular headaches.

High blood pressure can cause a common but dangerous type of vascular headache. Typically it is a dull pain that is felt all through the head. It is usually worse in the morning and lessens as the day progresses. People with this problem often find that the headache eases when they vomit.

It is just as important to note that most people with hypertension never develop headaches. The majority of hypertensive patients do not experience symptoms of any kind unless their high blood pressure has damaged internal organs such as the kidneys, heart, or brain. Have your blood pressure checked regularly. *If you have hypertension, don't wait to have symptoms before you start taking proper care of your problem.*

While nonprescription drugs can be very useful for headaches from hangover, caffeine withdrawal, and mild fever, a person who experiences any other type of vascular headache should see a doctor for treatment.

Sinus Headache

This type of headache differs from the others in that the pain is located in the front of the head, particularly around and behind the eyes. The headache is usually accompanied by nasal congestion, and, as the name indicates, is caused by clogged sinuses.

Sinus headache is usually caused by an infection of one or more sinuses. While antibiotics afford specific treatment, decongestants and aspirin can give some temporary relief until you can see your doctor.

Psychogenic Headache

Don't get the idea that you have to be psychotic or at

least neurotic to get this type of headache. Headache can be caused by everyday feelings such as apprehension, anxiety, or depression. Social or marital stress can also induce headaches.

I once developed psychogenic headaches from a job I hated. As soon as I walked through the front door of the hospital my head started to throb. The day I resigned the headaches disappeared, and I haven't been back in that building since—nor have the headaches been back.

Arthritis

Arthritis is a common condition that many people try to self-medicate. While there are at least a dozen different types of arthritis, one of the most common and potentially damaging forms is rheumatoid arthritis.

Rheumatoid arthritis is a chronic disease characterized by an inflammation of the linings of the joints. The disease initially attacks small joints, particularly those in the hands, fingers, feet, toes, and wrists.

Interestingly, one of the most effective drugs in the treatment of this and other types of arthritic disorders is plain aspirin. Two factors limit successful self-treatment of arthritis, however.

The first limitation is that the pain and crippling aspects of rheumatoid arthritis can progress if treatment is not adequate. The second has to do with the characteristics of aspirin itself.

People with arthritis frequently have to use tremendously high doses of aspirin to control their symptoms. These doses are very close to those that cause serious side effects.

Because of the characteristics of both the disease and the drug used to treat it, I don't recommend that anyone try to self-medicate arthritis. It would be nice if television advertisers would recognize their responsibility in this matter and discontinue commercials urging people to treat themselves with "arthritis strength" products.

Aspirin is one of the oldest and most effective treatments for arthritis. However, anyone suffering from *any* type of arthritis should be seeing a doctor regularly.

Dental Pain—How to Handle a Toothache

The best way to treat a toothache is to visit your dentist promptly. Any other type of treatment is only temporary.

People often look to OTC's for aid and comfort from toothache. Others turn to old home remedies. Those who try to avoid the inevitable trip to the dentist often end up using clove oil applications to the sore tooth and gum.

Clove oil and its active ingredient, eugenol, have been used as toothache remedies for years. Interestingly, eugenol is a potent protein destroyer. When clove oil is applied directly to a tooth and the surrounding gum it is capable of causing even more decay in the bad tooth and of irritating or even eating into the gum.

In other words, don't put clove oil on your teeth or gums.

Some people apply local remedies like Anbesol, Numzit, and Orajel to a sore tooth. While these products are safe, the FDA advisory panel could not prove that they are effective.

Aspirin is probably as good a toothache remedy as you can buy over the counter. However, when you use aspirin for a toothache you have to *swallow* the tablet. Some people make the mistake of placing the aspirin tablet directly on the sore tooth or gum and letting it dissolve there.

That's a bad idea.

First of all, aspirin can't relieve pain when it is placed directly on a painful area; it isn't an anesthetic. Secondly, when aspirin gets wet it breaks down into a strong acid that can destroy the enamel on your teeth. It can also cause nasty acid burns on the gums. Aspirin in the tummy works a lot better for your sore tooth than placing it directly on the tooth.

When You Have a Fever

Your body temperature is controlled by the hypothalamus, a bundle of nerve cells located near the base of your brain. This "thermostat" maintains your body temperature within one degree of its normal temperature.

This is a vital function because a body temperature higher than 106 degrees begins to fry the brain. Body temperatures greater than 110 degrees can cause brain death within a few hours.

The main mechanism that your body uses to get rid of excess heat is to increase the blood flow to your skin. This allows your body to radiate heat away from itself and into the surrounding room air. The drugs that we commonly use to treat fever work the same way.

Fever is another warning sign that there is something wrong in your body. While there are drugs that can reduce fever, they don't correct the underlying problem. Treating the fever is usually less important than finding and correcting its cause.

Most people assume that only infections cause fever. Actually, fever can result from allergic reactions, side effects of drugs, dehydration, and even some types of cancer. A fever that hangs on for several days can be an indication that something is seriously wrong and that a call to the doctor is needed.

Some Causes of Fever

Arthritis	Infection
Aspirin overdose	Mediterranean fever
Cancer	Pulmonary embolus
Crohn's disease	Rheumatic fever
Drug fever	Sarcoidosis
Fabry's disease	Systemic lupus
High blood cholesterol	erythematosus
levels	Thermoregulatory disorders

Internal Analgesics for Aches, Pain, and Fever

Internal analgesics are those wondrous little tablets and capsules that are able to relieve so many of our aches and pains. Those that are available over the counter can also reduce fever. Therefore, if you have the flu, headache, fever, and aching muscles, you can kill a whole flock of birds with one tablet.

There are three basic types of nonprescription pain relievers/fever reducers:

- The group known as the salicylates
- The well-advertised "non-aspirin" pain reliever acetaminophen
- The newest of the group, ibuprofen

We'll look at them in order of age, taking the salicylates first.

Salicylates—Aspirin and Its Cousins

The salicylates comprise a class of drugs chemically derived from salicylic acid. Aspirin is the best known and most commonly used drug of the group. All of the salicylates currently on the market have similar characteristics and can be considered together. Later on we'll look at some of the differences among the individual drugs in the group. For now, let's assume that they all do basically the same thing.

Until a few years ago we didn't have the foggiest idea of how aspirin worked. While we still have more questions than answers, some of the fog has lifted.

Now we know that pain-producing chemicals are released at the site of an injury or in response to a disease. These chemicals, known as prostaglandins, are present all over the body and are needed for many of the body's normal activities.

Aspirin decreases the body's ability to produce prostaglandins. This accounts for its pain-relieving (analgesic) effects. Aspirin is an efficient prostaglandin antagonist, which explains why the drug works so well for mild pain.

Prostaglandins are also partly responsible for the inflammation in some types of arthritis. When used properly, aspirin can be the best drug available for treating many cases of arthritis. However, as noted previously, arthritis should always be treated by a doctor.

Aspirin is one of the most effective prostaglandin inhibitors we have. However, prostaglandins aren't all bad.

Prostaglandins are chemical regulators in our bodies. Sometimes they get out of kilter, as in the cases of arthritis and menstrual cramps, and need to be put in their place. On the other hand, drugs that attack prostaglandins cause some serious side effects. For instance, prostaglandins protect our stomach linings from being dissolved by our own stomach acid. Aspirin and other drugs that hinder this prostaglandin effect can cause upset stomach and even ulcers. (We'll get to other side effects in a moment.)

Aspirin and the other salicylates are most effective in controlling the dull, aching type of pain, such as that felt from tension headache. They don't do much for sharp pains. If you smash your thumb doing some weekend carpentry, an aspirin won't be much help.

The salicylates are also effective antipyretics, or fever reducers. They complement the body's normal means of lowering temperature. In other words, they help the body carry out the brain's message to dilate the blood vessels in the skin. This vasodilation allows the body to get rid of excess heat. Fortunately, the salicylates don't cause people with normal body temperatures to lose heat.

Earlier I said that all the salicylates are virtually identical. Although the television hucksters won't tell you this, all of the salicylates, including aspirin and that "special" one you can only get in Doan's Pills, are converted to salicylic acid in the body!

Isn't that amazing? In spite of all the air time and money spent advertising these special formulas, they all turn into the same thing in your body.

Their most common side effect is stomach irritation. This is one of the few areas where there is some difference among the various salicylates.

Back in the nineteenth century and even into the twentieth century salicylic acid was a commonly used analgesic. However, salicylic acid is extremely irritating to the stomach and the rest of the gastrointestinal tract. Fortunately, it was found that aspirin caused significantly fewer problems of this type.

The salicylates are capable of causing any or all of these side effects:

- Bloody or black, tarlike stools
- Blurred vision

- Buzzing or a ringing sound in the ears
- Confusion
- Diarrhea
- Dizziness
- Headache or worsening of headache
- Impaired hearing
- Indigestion
- Rapid breathing
- Shortness of breath
- Stomach pain
- Sweating
- Thirst
- Tightness in the chest
- Vomiting
- Wheezing

Aspirin and Your Stomach

Heartburn and other forms of gastric pain and distress occur in 5 percent of all people who take aspirin, and the aspirin doesn't even need to pass through the stomach to do its number. Intravenous injections of aspirin have the same effect on the stomach as swallowing tablets!

Between 30 and 40 percent of all hospital admissions for bleeding ulcers are caused in part by salicylates. Some mild form of stomach bleeding occurs in more than half of all people who take aspirin.

This bleeding is no problem for most people. On the other hand, taking large doses of aspirin every day for months or years can cause enough blood loss to produce anemia.

Don't take aspirin or any other salicylate if you have or ever have had a peptic ulcer or any other type of stomach or intestinal bleeding. It isn't worth taking the risk that the drug could reactivate an old problem.

Many folks make a habit of taking a couple of aspirins or Alka-Seltzers for a hangover. That isn't such a good idea when you consider that the alcohol that caused the hangover also tears up your stomach. Putting aspirin down there can keep things churned up for some time. Aspirin can help your headache, but it can also do a number on your plumbing.

Aspirin and Your Blood

Aspirin also interferes with the function of platelets, the blood cells that control bleeding. Interestingly, aspirin seems to be the only salicylate that causes this effect.

Aspirin-induced inhibition of platelets is an obvious problem for some people with blood diseases. People who have diseases that predispose them to bleeding and those who take medications that alter their ability to clot blood should not take aspirin or any commercial product that contains aspirin. I have seen too many people develop near-fatal bleeding episodes due to this problem.

Those who have just had or are about to have surgery or dental procedures may also have some problems with aspirin. We know, for instance, that children who take aspirin immediately before or after they have their tonsils removed lose more blood than they should. We also know that aspirin causes blood to ooze for hours after a tooth extraction.

The effects of aspirin on the blood last a long time. In a normal, healthy person, one dose of two regular strength aspirin tablets affects clotting for as long as seven days. Therefore, it's important to avoid aspirin for at least a week before surgery or a dental visit.

On the other hand, it now appears that a small dose of aspirin taken each day can decrease your chances of having a heart attack or stroke!

If you are wondering how this can be, it really isn't too hard to figure out. Aspirin inhibits clumping of platelets and normal blood clotting, making it harder for clots to form in places they shouldn't be. Therefore, taking a small amount of aspirin can mean there is less likelihood of dangerous clots forming and then breaking away and lodging in vital blood vessels in the heart and brain.

The most effective dose for this purpose is just one children's aspirin (1¼ grains) per day. It doesn't seem to help to take more.

Allergies to Aspirin and the Salicylates

Like most drugs, aspirin and the salicylates can also cause allergic reactions. These reactions may appear in two forms.

The most common type of aspirin-induced allergic reaction is a form of asthma. This reaction is more common in women than men, and is more apt to occur after age fifty. Symptoms are identical to those of other types of asthma, with wheezing and difficulty exhaling air from the lungs. When it occurs, the reaction usually begins immediately after a dose of aspirin, but it can be delayed for as long as two hours.

If you have this problem, it is important to remember that aspirin in any form can cause this reaction. I once had a patient who knew she was allergic to aspirin but took a Darvon Compound capsule for her headache. Darvon Compound is a prescription drug that contains aspirin as one of its ingredients. Taking that one dose of Darvon Compound was enough to land her in the hospital with a severe asthma attack.

The second type of allergic reaction to aspirin is more characteristic of what we normally think of as an allergy. Symptoms include skin rash, hives, itching, and swelling. Of course, if you have one of these reactions you may also experience an asthma attack on top of this.

The most important lesson for those who are aspirin-allergic is to *read labels*. If you are allergic to aspirin (or anything else), be sure to read the label on the drug product you intend to buy. If in doubt about any of the ingredients, ask your pharmacist for advice.

While aspirin should not be taken during pregnancy, especially in the last few weeks before delivery, the reason isn't what you would suspect.

Remember the prostaglandins? The prostaglandin that causes menstrual cramps is also the one that is responsible for labor. Taking a prostaglandin inhibitor like aspirin delays the beginning of labor and lengthens the time it takes to deliver. That is not welcome news to Mom!

A second undesirable effect of aspirin taken as long as a week before delivery can increase the mother's blood loss and may interfere with blood clotting in the baby.

When You Should *Not* Use Aspirin

Don't try to use aspirin or any other salicylates if you have
any of these conditions:
  Alcohol hangover
  Any bleeding condition
  Aspirin allergy
  Iron deficiency anemia
  Stomach or intestinal ulcers
  If you know you are going to have surgery within one week
  If you are pregnant

If you have any doubt about whether or not any of this applies to you, talk to your pharmacist or doctor.

Aspirin Dosages

Aspirin would be a lot safer and a lot less confusing if
it were sold in standard dosage units. The usual adult dose
of aspirin for treating pain or fever is one or two 325-
milligram tablets every four hours while symptoms per-
sist. The maximum safe and effective adult single dose is
975 milligrams, or three regular strength tablets. Check
product labels for children's doses.

Since there are so many aspirin products on the market,
all trying to look a little different from the others, it may
be hard for you to find "standard strength" aspirin. Your
best bet is to buy plain label or store brand aspirin in the
325-milligram or 5-grain strength. You'll save yourself a
lot of confusion, not to mention money.

Be sure of the milligram strength of your tablets and
read label directions before you take aspirin. Some companies sell 20-grain (1300-milligram) aspirin tablets that
are intended to be taken only twice a day. You could poison yourself if you accidentally take two of these every
four hours.

Even familiar products like Anacin can cause problems
if you aren't careful. Remember, Anacin has more of that
ingredient doctors recommend most (aspirin). Two Anacin

tablets put you close to the maximum single dose of aspirin, and three tablets put you over the top.

One final word about the effectiveness of aspirin. A study of postoperative patients at the Mayo Clinic showed that two aspirin tablets were more effective in treating patients' pain than were the prescription drugs codeine, Darvon, or Talwin.

Aspirin Poisoning and Drug Interactions

Aspirin used to be the Number One culprit in childhood poisonings. This is no longer the case, since the arrival of those frustrating safety caps that you now find on your medicine bottles.

Aspirin poisoning is extremely dangerous in children. One of the problems is that toxic doses can produce fever and sweating. If parents don't know about the overdose, they may give even more aspirin to treat the fever. Early symptoms of aspirin poisoning include ringing or buzzing in the ears, difficulty hearing, nausea, vomiting, and diarrhea. Later the child may become confused and lapse into a coma.

The good news about aspirin poisoning is that it can be successfully treated if caught early enough. *If you have any doubt about whether a child has taken an overdose of aspirin, call your doctor or poison control center immediately.*

Another potential hazard of aspirin is its ability to interact with a large number of other drugs, including those listed below.

Drugs That Interact with Aspirin

Alcohol
Antidiabetic drugs
   Acetohexamide (Dymelor)
   Chlorpropamide (Diabinese)
   Tolazamide (Tolinase)
   Tolbutamide (Orinase)
Ascorbic acid (vitamin C)
Corticosteroids

    Dexamethasone (Decadron, Hexadrol)
    Methylprednisolone (Medrol)
    Prednisone (Deltasone, Orasone)
Heparin
Nonsteroidal anti-inflammatory drugs
    Fenoprofen (Nalfon)
    Ibuprofen (Motrin, Rufen)
    Indomethacin (Indocin)
    Ketoprofen (Orudis)
    Meclofenamate (Meclomen)
    Naproxen (Anaprox, Naprosyn)
    Phenylbutazone (Butazolidin)
    Sulindac (Clinoril)
    Tolmetin (Tolectin)
Methotrexate
Probenecid (Benemid)
Sulfinpyrazone (Anturane)
Warfarin (Coumadin)

Check with your pharmacist or doctor about the advisability of taking any of these drugs with aspirin or other salicylates.

Forms of Aspirin Commercially Available

Aspirin and the other salicylates are commercially available in a dazzling assortment of colors, shapes, and sizes. Thanks to American ingenuity, you can buy aspirin and its counterparts in:

- Buffered tablets
- Capsules
- Chewable tablets
- Chewing gum
- Effervescent solutions
- Enteric coated tablets
- Micronized particles
- Plain tablets
- Powders
- Suppositories
- Sustained-release tablets

Of all the types of products listed above, the only two that I normally recommend are plain aspirin tablets and children's chewable tablets. Any slight advantage any of the other formulations may have to offer is more than offset by its price.

Different Forms of Aspirin

Aspirin Tablets

It has not been proven that one brand of plain aspirin is consistently better than another.

Examples: Aspirin USP, Bayer Aspirin

Buffered Tablets

These contain a small amount of antacid, supposedly to protect the stomach from aspirin's irritating effects. Buffers do not produce a meaningful decrease in stomach acidity nor do they protect the stomach from aspirin's effects.

Examples: Ascriptin, Ascriptin A/D, Bufferin

Effervescent Solutions

These solutions are made by dropping effervescent tablets in water. A chemical reaction between an acid and a base takes place and the solution fizzes. The reaction produces an aspirin solution that has not been shown to be more effective than an equivalent dose of aspirin tablets.

Example: Alka-Seltzer

Enteric Coated Tablets

These are supposed to dissolve in the intestine rather than the stomach. Unfortunately, the absorption of aspirin from these tablets is unpredictable. They offer no special advantages over plain tablets.

Examples: ASA Enseal, Ecotrin

Capsules

Some people find capsules to be easier to swallow than tablets.

Example: ASA Pulvules

Sustained-Release Tablets

These offer the convenience of less frequent dosing; however, the aspirin in these tablets is not completely absorbed from the gastrointestinal tract.

Examples: Bayer Timed Release Aspirin, Measurin

Chewable Tablets

These are intended for small children, who need smaller doses than older children and adults and often cannot swallow tablets.

Examples: Bayer Children's Aspirin, St. Joseph's Aspirin for Children

Powders

Powders are commonly used in some areas, particularly in the South. They offer no advantage over aspirin tablets except for those who cannot swallow a tablet or capsule. They have the disadvantages of expense and bad taste.

Examples: BC Powder, Stanback Powder

Chewing Gum

Gums are less effective and much more expensive than aspirin tablets. Only the portion of the aspirin that leaves the gum and is swallowed is effective. Aspirin chewing gums also expose the teeth, gums, and throat to the corrosive effects of aspirin.

Example: Aspergum

Suppositories

Suppositories should only be used if giving aspirin is absolutely essential and there is no other way of administering a dose. Suppositories can irritate and inflame the rectum and their absorption is unreliable.

Aspirin in Combination with Other Drugs

As if developing and marketing a batch of superfluous types of aspirin products were not enough, our drug companies have provided us with a cornucopia of combinations of aspirin with analgesics and other drugs that have little or nothing to do with pain relief. Some of the products that I find most offensive are Alka-Seltzer, Bufferin, Anacin, and Excedrin.

While Alka-Seltzer has been soundly criticized by health professionals for years, the public continues to buy it. Did you know that two Alka-Seltzer tablets contain 1042 milligrams of sodium? A single dose of two tablets is equivalent to more salt than some people are allowed in their diet for a whole day!

Some people use Alka-Seltzer as an antacid. The problem is that the drug contains aspirin, which can irritate the stomach and even worsen an ulcer. Given that fact, it doesn't seem to make much sense to use it as an antacid, does it?

The practice of polypharmacy, the use of combinations of drugs when one will do, is alive and well as far as nonprescription analgesics are concerned. Combinations are more common than single drug products. A good example is Anacin.

You remember Anacin, the drug that has "more of the drug doctors recommend most," plus an extra ingredient. Anacin contains 400 milligrams of the ingredient doctors actually do recommend most, aspirin, while plain aspirin tablets usually have the standard 325 milligrams. And that "special ingredient"? It's just a small amount of caffeine.

Combination Products and Kidney Problems

A really bizarre, long-term side effect of pain-killers is a condition known as analgesic nephropathy. Fortunately, this potentially fatal complication is seen in very few people in the United States, although it is common in some other countries. It is the most common cause of kidney failure in Sweden and Australia.

Analgesic nephropathy is a disease apparently caused by the continuous heavy use of analgesic *combination* products for periods of years at a time. The current medical opinion is that aspirin taken alone rarely causes this condition. Rather, the combination of aspirin and the analgesic phenacetin is the main culprit.

It is interesting that experiments using phenacetin by

itself were not able to cause kidney disease. The problem seems to be related to the concurrent use of phenacetin with something else. If you have been accustomed to using APC (aspirin, phenacetin, and caffeine) tablets for your aches and pains, you may notice that the product is no longer available.

It seems to me that phenacetin has gotten a bum rap. The drug appears to be safe when used by itself and most of the evidence against it is purely circumstantial. Ironically, it now appears that the *combination of aspirin and acetaminophen,* if taken in high doses for long enough, may also induce analgesic nephropathy.

Who in the world would take such a combination? I doubt that too many people would intentionally dose up with both of these drugs, but some products do contain this combination. Excedrin tablets and capsules are examples, and so are the generic copies you can find in many drug and grocery stores.

The good news about analgesic nephropathy is that it is extremely rare if you only take occasional doses of aspirin or acetaminophen. It is also rare even if you take high doses of aspirin for long periods of time, as is the case for many people with arthritis, as long as you take plain aspirin.

Other Types of Salicylates

I mentioned earlier that there are several other salicylates, or aspirinlike drugs, on the market. The more common ones are aluminum aspirin, sodium salicylate, magnesium salicylate, choline salicylate, and calcium carbaspirin.

Don't let advertising fool you. None of these has any significant advantage over aspirin, with the possible exception of choline salicylate. This is the only salicylate that is chemically stable in water, and its advantage is that it can be used in liquid preparations. Anthropan is the best-known product containing choline salicylate.

Salicylamide is sometimes referred to as a "nonsalicylate" salicylate. Its effects are identical to the salicylates, but it doesn't break down to salicylic acid when it is absorbed into the blood.

The main problem with salicylamide is that it is easily destroyed by enzymes in the intestines and liver. You have to take at least 600 milligrams for it to reach the bloodstream. In addition to not working as well as aspirin, even if you take enough, an average adult's liver destroys half of the amount absorbed within one hour.

Products that contain salicylamide include Arthralgen, Bancap, Banesin, Cystex, DeWitt Pills, Meadache, Panodynes Analgesic, Rid-A-Pain, and Stanback Powder.

Acetaminophen—A Possible Alternative to Aspirin

Acetaminophen, whose best-known brand name is Tylenol, was developed as an alternative to aspirin. It has about the same effects on pain and fever as aspirin but doesn't cause the stomach upset or bleeding that can occur with aspirin.

For many patients acetaminophen is a satisfactory alternative to aspirin. It's easier on the stomach than aspirin and it doesn't affect blood clotting. Acetaminophen is an excellent choice for people who need something to relieve pain from minor surgery or dental procedures. It can also be used safely by people who are allergic to aspirin.

But before you begin to think that acetaminophen is the perfect analgesic, be aware that it has two important differences from aspirin. The first is a disappointment; the second is deadly.

Acetaminophen has no effect on inflammatory processes. Therefore, it has only limited effectiveness in treating arthritis.

The more important distinction from aspirin is that *acetaminophen overdoses are extremely dangerous*.

Overdoses of acetaminophen destroy the liver and must be treated *immediately* after the overdose has occurred. One of the problems is that the victim usually feels fine for as long as two days after the poisoning. If you or someone you know waits for symptoms to start to get medical attention, there is a good chance that nothing can be done.

Only in the last few years has an effective treatment for acetaminophen overdose been known. When I managed a poison control center in the early 1970s I had to watch a little girl die of a Tylenol overdose because we didn't know of any effective treatments at that time.

If you have small children in your home, if you have small grandchildren, or if small children come into your house on occasion, please keep your Tylenol or other brand of acetaminophen out of reach and in a child-resistant container. Children continue to die of these poisonings because adults don't know that the drug is dangerous.

It doesn't require a lot of acetaminophen to cause problems. A dose as low as thirty Extra-Strength Tylenol or Anacin-3 tablets can kill an adult. As few as ten can kill a child.

Those who take acetaminophen daily also have cause for concern. Acetaminophen is classified as a "predictable" liver toxin. There are some specialists who believe that long-term use of normal doses of acetaminophen can produce liver problems.

This is not to say that there is no use for the drug. Acetaminophen is safe at recommended doses; I use it myself instead of aspirin. But I don't believe that there is any need for the "extra strength" forms. They are usually more expensive, contain more medication than is needed, and are frequently implicated in accidental overdoses.

Acetaminophen is available in store brands or as plain-label tablets and capsules. You don't need to spend extra money on the nationally advertised brands.

Remember also that the combination of aspirin and acetaminophen can lead to kidney disease if the two are taken in combination for long periods of time. In addition, there is no advantage to taking the two drugs together. The combination is no better than either drug taken alone in an adequate dose.

Some brands of aspirin-acetaminophen combinations are BC Tablets and Powders, Capron, Excedrin, Excedrin P.M., Goody's Tablets and Powders, Trigesic, and Vanquish.

Ibuprofen—A Recent OTC Formulation

Ibuprofen is the new kid on the analgesic block.

Ibuprofen was originally available by prescription only. When the FDA allowed it to be released in 1984 for over-the-counter sale, it was the fifth most commonly prescribed drug in America and was being taken by almost 7 million people in this country alone.

The higher strengths of ibuprofen are still restricted to prescription status and are sold under the brand names Motrin and Rufen. The OTC tablets contain only 200 milligrams and are available as Advil and Nuprin.

Ibuprofen is effective for the relief of minor aches and pains associated with the common cold, headache, toothache, muscle aches, backache, menstrual cramps, and for reduction of fever. In other words, it can be used for the same conditions as aspirin or acetaminophen.

The usual dose of ibuprofen is one 200-milligram tablet every four to six hours as needed for relief of symptoms. You may take two tablets at a time, but the chances of side effects rise considerably if you do this. Don't take more than six tablets in a day without consulting your pharmacist or doctor.

The drug has not been adequately tested in children. Don't give it to anyone less than twelve years old unless so directed by a pediatrician. It has also been associated with some birth defects when taken during pregnancy.

Unlike acetaminophen, ibuprofen is *not safe* for people who are allergic to aspirin. If you have an aspirin allergy you may experience the same reaction with ibuprofen. Even though the two drugs are chemically dissimilar, the body's immune system can't tell the difference between the two.

The frequency of side effects with ibuprofen is low, but they do occur. If you experience any of these symptoms while taking ibuprofen, see your doctor immediately:

- Black or bloody stools
- Blood in the urine
- Changes in vision
- Dark colored urine
- Frequent urge to urinate
- Ringing or buzzing in the ears
- Swelling of the feet or legs
- Tarlike stools
- Tightness or pain in the chest
- Unexplained sore throat or fever

- Pain with urination
- Rash, hives, or itching
- Wheezing or shortness of breath

These side effects occur in fewer than 1 percent of all people who take ibuprofen. However, if they happen, they can indicate serious problems and their presence should not be ignored.

About 10 percent of people experience one or more of the following side effects when taking ibuprofen. These effects are more of a nuisance than a danger. If they occur and are bothersome to you, consult your pharmacist or doctor for advice.

- Bloated feeling
- Diarrhea or constipation
- Dizziness
- Gas
- Headache
- Heartburn or indigestion
- Loss of appetite
- Nausea or vomiting
- Nervousness

Ibuprofen has no particular advantages or disadvantages when compared to aspirin or acetaminophen. It's simply different. You can try using ibuprofen if you like, but you will probably get about the same response you would have had from one of the other, cheaper drugs.

Muscle Aches

Most muscle aches are characterized by pain and stiffness, often of sudden onset. They occur most frequently in the neck, shoulders, and lower back. Back pain and spasms can also extend into the buttocks and down the legs.

Lifting heavy loads, poor posture, and obesity are common causes of muscle pain. Pain can be caused by strains and sprains, nonarthritic rheumatic conditions, and strenuous exercise. Stiffness and pain can also result from exposure to cold and dampness, rapid temperature changes, bruises, and immobilization, such as when driving a car long distances.

Strains and sprains cause similar types of pain, but actually are very different. A *strain* results from stress or injury to a muscle. A *sprain* is an injury to a joint or to the ligaments around a joint. Sprains are much more serious than strains and should never be self-treated.

Muscle pains that last longer than a week should be evaluated by a doctor or physical therapist. Pain that doesn't go away in a few days can indicate a sprain, fracture, arthritis, or other serious disease state. For instance, in many people the first symptom of a urinary tract infection is a backache.

Arthritis, as noted, should never be self-treated. While there are OTC remedies that are effective for treating arthritis, some may allow the disease to progress. *There is no substitute for a doctor's supervision in arthritis.*

Topical Analgesics—Relief Through Counter-Irritation

People often look toward topical analgesic ointments, creams, gels, sticks, aerosols, and lotions for relief of muscle pain. It seems to make sense that applying a medication directly over a painful spot should help to relieve the pain. I have little doubt that the use of counter-irritants has a strong psychological component and that placebo effects probably play a major role in the effectiveness of all of these drugs.

These products are not without drawbacks. Many people assume them to be completely safe since they are applied outside the body. In reality, any medication applied to the skin can be absorbed into the blood and cause systemic side effects. In fact, some drugs, like Aspercreme, have to be absorbed in order to work.

Most of the ingredients in these products are counter-irritants. In other words, they work by irritating the skin. The theory is that they cause the nerves in the skin to transmit a feeling of heat or coolness. When these nerve impulses go to the brain they interfere with the painful impulses from the muscle. In the end, the brain only receives the impulses from the skin surface because the painful impulses from the muscle are blocked. This is part of the gate control theory of pain.

If these drugs are irritants to the skin, what do you think they do if you use too much?

You don't have to be a pharmacologic genius to guess— they can cause rashes, blisters, burns, and even skin ulcers. Some of the newer ''odorless' products may be more likely to do this than the older ones, since people find the newer ones to be less objectionable and therefore may overuse them.

If you find that you have applied too much, you can usually remove most of it with a cotton cloth or gauze pad soaked in vegetable oil. Be sure you also wash your hands thoroughly after each application, because leftovers may sting your hands. Also, be sure not to get any under your rings or other jewelry or you'll swear your finger is on fire.

Counter-irritants, topical analgesics, or whatever you want to call them have been a part of folk medicine for centuries. Unfortunately, we still aren't sure of exactly how they work or even if they work. Some experts feel that any beneficial effects derived from counter-irritants may simply be due to rubbing and massaging the drug back into the skin.

Types of Counter-Irritants

Many counter-irritants can be found on the OTC market. Unfortunately, the FDA advisory panel examining these drugs did not apply very strict standards to them. Consequently, many are still on the market that don't deserve to be there.

The panel also allowed products to remain on the market even if their manufacturers were not able to prove that all their ingredients were effective. Some approved products have as many as five ''active'' ingredients.

There is no advantage to combinations of these drugs. If you use a combination product, how do you know which ingredient is working or which is causing side effects? Often the price of a product is directly proportional to the number of ingredients. This is a shame, because an adequate concentration of one of these drugs is every bit as good as a combination.

Many of these combinations are totally irrational. For instance, some contain local anesthetics or skin protectants with the counter-irritant. These additives cancel the effect of the irritant. Some examples of these types of combinations are Analgesic Balm, Exocaine Plus, Icy Hot, Mentholatum Deep Heeting, Minit-Rub, and Panalgesic.

The box below provides you with a list of the most common counter-irritants and some comments about each of them.

Ingredients Found in Topical Analgesics

Camphor

Its pleasant smell and the feeling of coolness it produces make camphor a popular ingredient in analgesics.

Warning: Camphorated oil is sometimes mistaken for castor oil and taken internally. Accidental camphor ingestions are always serious. Less than two teaspoonfuls of camphorated oil can be fatal to an adult.

Menthol

This extract of peppermint oil is often combined with camphor. In low concentrations menthol relieves itching and in higher amounts acts as a counter-irritant. Menthol can cause rashes, hives, and severe reddening of the skin.

Turpentine Oil

This mainstay of American folk remedies causes allergic reactions in up to 10 percent of the people who use it. Applying turpentine oil to the skin may cause blisters, hives, and vomiting in susceptible people. Pharmaceutical grade turpentine oil is of higher quality than the commercial grade.

Capsicum

This is one of the few counter-irritants that does not cause blistering, even in high concentrations.

Methyl Nicotinate

Methyl nicotinate is a derivative of the B vitamin niacin. The drug penetrates the skin rapidly and, when applied over large areas on susceptible people, can drop the blood pressure and the heart rate.

Methyl Salicylate

Oil of wintergreen or sweet birch oil are common synonyms for methyl salicylate. It is the most commonly used counter-irritant and is also one of the most deadly if taken orally by accident. Less than a teaspoonful can kill a small child.

Triethanolamine Salicylate

This drug does not work on the skin the way the other counter-irritants do. It must be absorbed through the skin and into the blood in order to work. There are some data indicating that some of it actually is absorbed, but probably not enough to relieve muscle or joint pain. One evaluation of the drug in patients with degenerative arthritis showed that it was no more effective than a nonmedicated ointment. If triethanolamine salicylate must be absorbed into the blood to be effective, why not just take an aspirin tablet? Triethanolamine salicylate is the "active" ingredient in Aspercreme and Mobisyl.

Use Caution with Counter-Irritants

It is important to remember that, although counter-irritants are used outside the body, they can cause serious problems. The following story is an example.

A three-year-old girl with epileptic-like seizures was brought to a hospital emergency room. Her mother told the hospital staff that she had been treating the girl's drippy nose by shoving Vicks Vaporub (4.81 percent camphor) up her daughter's nostrils twice a day for the last five months. Two hours before the first convulsion the mother saw the child with an open jar of Vaporub and it appeared that about one tablespoonful was missing. Since the girl enjoyed the taste of the stuff, the hospital staff correctly assumed that she had eaten the missing Vaporub.

Fortunately, this case turned out all right. Unfortunately, many others involving other camphor-containing preparations have not.

Camphor and some of the other ingredients in these products are deadly poisons. If you must keep these drugs in your house, be aware that children are often attracted to them. Some liniments and lotions look like milk or other treats. Children may also mistake creams like Ben-Gay for toothpaste.

Just because these products don't look like "medicine" does not mean that you should not treat them as such.

Topical analgesics constitute a unique class of drugs in that absorption of their ingredients is not a desired property. Unfortunately, all of them are absorbed to some extent. Most of these products have the following warnings on their labels:

- For external use only.
- Avoid contact with eyes.
- If the condition worsens, discontinue the use of this product and consult a physician.
- Do not use on children under two except with the advice and under the supervision of a physician.
- Do not apply to wounds or damaged skin.
- Do not bandage.

The manufacturers of these products aren't kidding when they list these warnings. Even on healthy skin, the margin of safety with these drugs can be thin. Stop using these preparations if excessive skin irritation develops.

Believe me, the skin problems these drugs can cause can be much more serious than the original symptoms you were trying to treat.

I believe that you can get more pain relief from taking aspirin, acetaminophen, or ibuprofen by mouth than you can from any counter-irritant.

There is too much mysticism attached to these products. Their advertising doesn't help to clarify things either.

DMSO—Not for Medical Use!

One black market topical analgesic that certainly does work for some types of pain is dimethylsulfoxide, or DMSO. DMSO has been used to treat a variety of disorders, but most commonly for arthritis. A unique property of DMSO is its ability to cross through the skin and go into the blood. The problem is that it can also carry impurities into the blood with it.

DMSO has not been approved by the FDA for human use except for a rare bladder condition called interstitial cystitis. The only DMSO you can buy is chemical grade, not pharmaceutical grade. The chemical grade product may contain a wide variety of potentially dangerous contaminants. DMSO can pull these contaminants into the blood with it and cause a whole mess of potentially serious illnesses.

It never ceases to amaze me that some people will slop on the local hardware store's DMSO without giving a second thought to the dangers and yet grow livid over one part per billion of dioxin in dirt.

Do not use DMSO. It is dangerous and not worth the risk.

Besides the potential for poisoning with foreign substances, DMSO has its own side effects. The best known is the garlic breath it imparts to its users. The taste of garlic may last for several hours. The odor usually takes about three days to clear.

In addition, DMSO can cause severe allergic reactions, disturbances in color vision and visual acuity, cataracts, headache, nausea, diarrhea, rashes, and burning on urination. It also causes birth defects in animals.

Pfizer Consumer Products, makers of Ben-Gay, occasionally runs an ad stating that their product is effective in warming muscles prior to exercise. When I contacted Pfizer to request data supporting this claim, they responded that they cannot send copies of the clinical studies, as this information is "proprietary."

However, they did tell me that "Ben-Gay did not improve running efficiency."

꙳

The Pharmacist's Prescription for Pain and Fever

For aches and fever use plain-label or store brand aspirin or acetaminophen 325-milligram tablets for adults. Children may use acetaminophen chewable tablets or liquids or aspirin chewable tablets.

Aspirin, acetaminophen, or ibuprofen by mouth work as well for muscle pain as any of the topical analgesics. If these do not give sufficient pain relief, you can try applying heat by using a heat lamp, a hot water bottle, a heating pad, or a moist steam pack. Regulate the temperature to produce a warming sensation without causing a burn. *Do not apply heat if you are using a counter-irritant.*

See the Doctor if . . .
You have a fever and . . .
- Your temperature goes above 103°F or 39.5°C.
- Your fever lasts longer than three days.
- Your fever does not respond to medication.
- You have difficulty breathing.
- You have a sore throat.
- You have pain when you pass urine.

You have a headache and . . .
- Your headache causes extreme or incapacitating pain.
- Your headache is accompanied by stiff neck, fever, changes in vision, weakness, loss of feeling in any part of your body, confusion, or personality changes.

You have joint or muscle pain and . . .
- You have intense or sudden pain or swelling in a muscle or joint.
- You find that normal movements cause pain.
- Your joint pain is accompanied by a fever.
- You cannot move a joint.
- You have numbness or tingling in a joint or muscle.
- You have arthritis.

Products Recommended for Pain or Fever
Aspirin products
Bayer Aspirin
St. Joseph Aspirin

Ibuprofen
Doan's Ibuprofen Pills
Acetaminophen products
Haltran
Acetamin
Medipren
Datril
Midol 200
SK-APAP
Nuprin
Tylenol
Trendar

Or the generic equivalent of any of the above

Analgesics Not Recommended for Self-Medication
Internal medications
Alka-Seltzer (E,I)
Allerest Headache Strength (I)
Anacin (I)
Anacin, Maximum Strength (I)
APC (E,I)
Arthritis Pain Formula (H,I)
Arthritis Strength Bufferin (H,I)
ASA Compound (H,I)
Ascriptin (H,I)
Ascriptin A/D (H,I)
Aspergum (B)
BC Powder (I)
BC Tablets (I)
Bromo-Seltzer (E,I)
Bufferin (H,I)
Cama (H,I)
Congespirin (I)
Cope (I)
DeWitt Pills (I)
Doan's Pills (I)

Excedrin (I)
Excedrin P.M. (I)
Goody's Extra Strength Tablets (I)
Goody's Headache Powder (I)
Momentum (I)
PAC (I)
Percogesic(I)
Rid-A-Pain (I)
Sinarest (I)
Sine-Aid (I)
Trigesic (I)
Vanquish (H,I)
Topical medications
Absorbine Arthritic (D,I)
Absorbine Jr. (D,I)
Analgesic Balm (D,I)
Aspercreme (A)
Banalg (D,I)
Banalg Hospital Strength (D,I)
Ben-Gay (D,I)

Ben-Gay Extra Strength (D,I)
Ben-Gay Gel (D,I)
Ben-Gay Greaseless/ Stainless Ointment (D,I)
Ben-Gay Original (D,I)
Counterpain Rub (D,I)
Doan's Rub (D,I)
Exocaine Medicated Rub (D,I)
Exocaine Plus (D,I)
Heet (D,I)
Icy Hot (D,I)
Infra-Rub (D,I)

Mentholatum (D,I)
Mentholatum Deep Heating (D,I)
Minit-Rub (D,I)
Mobisyl (A)
Musterole (D,I)
Omega Oil (D,I)
Panalgesic (D,I)
Rid-A-Pain (D,I)
Sloan's Liniment (D,I)
Zemo Liquid (I)
Zemo Liquid Extra Strength (I)
Zemo Ointment (I)

Or the generic equivalent of any of the above

The products listed in the "Not Recommended" tables are not recommended by me for one or more of the following reasons: (A) One or more ingredients have been reported to be ineffective or only slightly effective for the product's intended purpose; (B) a more effective product is available; (C) the product advertising or description is likely to heighten consumer expectation beyond actual effectiveness; (D) the product has the potential to cause side effects in the average consumer that are more serious than those generally associated with OTC drugs; (E) the product has the potential to cause serious side effects in persons with specific diseases or disorders; (F) another product is available that is capable of producing the same or nearly the same therapeutic effect without the same risk of side effects; (G) persistent use of the product may cause physical dependency that alters an otherwise normal body function; (H) the product's formulation may reduce the effectiveness of one of its ingredients; (I) this is a multiple-ingredient product that may have no therapeutic advantage over simpler or single-ingredient products; (J) one or more of the product's ingredients may be useful for only a short period during the total duration of the illness; (K) the product cannot easily be administered at a dosage level within generally recommended boundaries of optimal therapeutic effect; (L) this is a condition-specific product that is appropriate for use only after a health professional has helped the patient establish a diagnosis.

4

Taking Care of Your Skin

It will never get well if you pick it.
—American Proverb

Skin is the largest and least appreciated organ of the body. Your skin is responsible for:

- Protecting underlying tissue from heat, sun, chemicals, and bacteria
- Preventing excess water loss
- Regulating body temperature by preventing loss of heat in winter and promoting heat loss in summer
- Storing reserve food and water
- Eliminating water and salts
- Protecting the body against the entry of foreign substances
- Detecting pleasurable or harmful stimuli

Skin, its subcomponents, and derivatives make up the integumentary system. Your body's oil glands, mammary glands, hair and hair follicles, and finger and toe nails are all part of this system.

The skin is formed into two layers. The epidermis, the outermost layer, is itself composed of four distinct layers. The dermis is positioned below the epidermis and contains blood vessels, oil glands, hair shafts, hair follicles, nerve fibers, sweat glands, and tough, fibrous connective tissue. In animals we use this skin layer to make leather.

Except for the stratum corneum, the top layer of the epidermis, all layers of the skin are living tissue and have to be supplied with oxygen, water, and nutrients. Most of the oxygen for the upper layers of skin is supplied by blood vessels in the lower layers.

Water is critical to the health of your skin. Since it is difficult to supply enough water to the epidermis, the skin must maintain its own system of water preservation. The sebaceous (oil) glands constantly secrete oily sebum to lubricate the skin surface and trap water inside the skin. If the epidermis becomes dehydrated, it loses elasticity, flakes off, becomes irritated, and allows infections to start. We'll cover this in more detail later in this chapter in the section on dry skin.

Since the skin is a living barrier, not a plastic wrapping, it has the potential to absorb substances that are placed on it. Depending upon the circumstances, this can be an advantage or disadvantage. In some cases, we apply medication to the skin in the hope that it will soak in and go either to a lower layer of skin or into the blood. In other cases, absorption of drugs through the skin can cause unanticipated side effects.

Throughout this chapter I will be referring to structures of the skin that may not be familiar to you. I've provided a glossary to help you with some of these terms.

Glossary of Dermatology Terms

Comedo. A blackhead or whitehead. A follicle that is plugged with sebum.

Dermis. The deepest layer of skin. Contains blood vessels, lymphatics, nerves, connective tissue, elastic fibers, and sweat and sebaceous glands.

Epidermis. The outermost portion of skin. Consists of four distinct layers.

Follicle. A small channel through the epidermis that allows the passage of sweat, sebum, and a hair shaft.

Sebaceous gland. The oil-secreting gland in the skin.

Sebum. The skin's natural oil. Secreted by the sebaceous glands.

Stratum corneum. The layer of dead cells on the surface

of the skin. The end product of the rest of the skin. Provides the skin's protective quality.

Acne—A Complex Disease

Acne is more than an attack on an adolescent's vanity. Severe acne can cause permanent scarring of both skin and psyche. There is no OTC *cure* for acne, but in the past decade we have learned considerably more than we knew before about its causes and treatment.

Treatment of acne can be long and costly. There are effective OTC treatments, but many of the nonprescription remedies on the market today are not worth bothering with.

Acne is a complex disease. The trouble starts deep inside the skin long before blotches and pimples appear on the face or other part of the body.

Normally the oil produced by the sebaceous glands rises to the top of the skin through the follicles that surround the hair shafts. The movement of sebum to the skin's surface is an important part of the skin's garbage disposal system. The cells lining the follicles are continually dying and being replaced, and as they die they slough off from the follicle walls and fall into the oil. For unknown reasons, some follicle cells begin to clump up and slow the flow of sebum. These clusters of cells and sebum mix with other skin materials, including pigments and bacteria, and form a plug below the surface of the skin. When the follicles get plugged, the sebum and dead cells accumulate and the real trouble starts. The plug acts as a dam, holding back sebum and its traveling companions. The result is a microcomedo, the beginning of an acne lesion.

The microcomedo lurks beneath the surface of the skin, and it may take several weeks before it bursts upon the scene. As the sebaceous gland continues to spout oil into the clogged system, pressure builds behind the dam and one of two things happens: (1) The oil plug may migrate to the surface of the skin and appear as a blackhead, more properly referred to as an ''open comedo''; or (2) the plug may stay below the surface, appearing as a whitehead, or ''closed comedo.''

Despite what your mother said, blackheads aren't caused by poor hygiene, lack of soap, or improper skin care. Blackheads originate below the skin (where soap can't reach) and turn black because they mix with skin pigments in the follicle, not dirt. Anyone can develop blackheads, no matter how often they wash.

Whiteheads are the real problem in acne. Since they can't get out via the top of the follicle, pressure continues to build and they eventually burst downward into the deeper layers of skin. The ruptured follicle spills its contents into the surrounding tissue and an inflammatory reaction begins. Inflammation causes pus to collect and the skin surface reddens. The reddened area is the pimple that we're all familiar with.

The life span of a single acne pimple is relatively short. It usually disappears by itself in about ten days. Almost everyone experiences a few of these episodes throughout life. In severe cases of acne, however, dozens of eruptions may be occurring simultaneously.

Continuous insults to the dermis and hypodermis from chronic acne can cause permanent pitting and scarring. Anyone who has severe inflammatory acne should be under a dermatologist's care to prevent severe cosmetic and emotional problems.

Acne, more properly called *acne vulgaris,* occurs most commonly on the face, chest, and back. It usually begins with puberty and is part of the skin's reaction to rising levels of the hormones testosterone and progesterone.

The chances of developing acne are greatest at age fourteen for girls and sixteen for boys. Cystic acne, the most damaging form, affects males more commonly than females. However, acne isn't limited to adolescents; acne can occur in small children and in middle-aged and older adults.

About 75 percent of teenagers have acne, and about 25 percent have moderate to severe cases. Only 10 percent of high school acne sufferers seek a doctor's help; 60 percent self-medicate. Moderate to severe acne is more common in white adolescents than in blacks of the same age. Mild acne is more common in blacks.

There are two basic types of acne, inflammatory and

noninflammatory. Noninflammatory acne is simply the tendency to form blackheads. Most people don't realize that this is acne.

Inflammatory acne is a more serious problem. This consists of what we typically consider to be acne—blemishes, blotches, inflammation, and pimples. In bad cases permanent cysts, scars, and pits can form. Fortunately, Accutane, a new prescription medication, limits some of the damage.

Since even moderate cases of inflammatory acne can result in scars, you should see a dermatologist rather than attempt self-treatment.

Aggravating Factors in Acne

Getting your first pimple isn't bad enough. We also have to deal with folklore about the causes and cures of these skin eruptions.

Take the old admonishment to avoid candy and chocolate. The truth is that foods don't cause acne. They don't make it worse either. The only consistent association between rashes, sugar, chocolate, and other confections is that people who are sensitive to them may have *allergic* reactions on the face and other areas. In some cases, these reactions may be mistaken for acne.

The same is true of greasy foods. You can still enjoy a Big Mac and a chocolate milk shake. They may be tough on your waistline, but they won't make your face worse.

If sweets and grease don't make your acne flare up, what does?

Unfortunately, the most important aggravating factors are unavoidable. Your normal hormone surge is the trigger for acne formation. It's no accident that acne begins at puberty, when your hormones kick in. About two-thirds of women with acne have a hormone-related flare-up just before their menstrual periods begin.

Stress also contributes to acne. Why does acne always seem to get worse just before a big date? Anxiety and emotional stress cause the release of another hormone, cortisol, which seems to aggravate the skin.

Stress may arise from different sources. Trouble at home or in school, money problems, even worrying about an uncertain future can make a teenager's face look like raw meat. Actually, the only link between eating chocolate and new acne sores is the fact that teens often *worry* that they'll get more pimples because they ate something they didn't think they should.

Sometimes the very things we use to treat or cover pimples can make them worse.

One of the biggest problems girls and women have is the facial makeup they use. Some makeup can clog healthy pores and create new pimples. "Cleansers" like cold cream and products that have similar consistency do the same job on your skin. Even hair dressings that contain oil can cause acne at the hairline.

If you have to use makeup, try to use hypoallergenic brands. Most women seem to tolerate these better. If the label says that the product is oil-free, that's all the better.

Irritation to the skin can also inflame and worsen acne sores. Unfortunately, it doesn't take much irritation to do this.

Although it is important to keep your skin clean, vigorous scrubbing, excessive washing, and the overuse of abrasive acne skin cleansers can make your condition worse. Remember that your skin is a delicate organ. While you must keep your skin clean, overdoing things can cause more trouble than you started with.

Skin trauma is not limited to washing. You can also irritate your skin by wearing rough clothing, headbands, or other types of athletic equipment or clothing. The chin strap on a football helmet is a good example.

Don't scratch or pick at your skin. You'll only make matters worse. Even a habit as simple as resting your chin on your hand during class can irritate your skin.

But avoiding acne can only go so far. What can you do to treat the pimples you have already?

Treating Acne

When you walk into the pharmacy, you seem to be accosted by rows and rows of acne products. How do you choose from among the soaps, creams, cleansers, peeling agents, cover-ups, lotions, gels, pads, and whatever the newest miracle product happens to be?

There's good news for acne-sufferers. Chances are that with the help of over-the-counter products you can *reduce* the number and severity of your pimples. The bad news is that there is no OTC *cure* for acne.

There is no quick solution to your acne problem. Treatment has to be prolonged and consistent. If you're a teenager, you will probably have to treat your condition for months, even years, before you grow out of it. If you're an adult with acne, you may have it for the rest of your life.

The basic principles in acne treatment are simple. All you have to do is:

- Remove excess skin oil.
- Prevent oil ducts from closing.
- Minimize stress and skin damage.
- Control your hormone flow.
- Stop using cosmetics.

Unfortunately, it is impossible to do all those things.

So where do you go from here? All acne products sound good when they are advertised on television. Should you just go to the drugstore, buy one of each type, rush home, and slop it all on in hopes that something works?

Of course not!

If we look at the ingredients of some of the common OTC acne aids, we'll find that some of the ingredients are antiques. Drugs like alcohol, resorcinol, sulfur, and salicylic acid have been around forever. They probably all work, but a newer product is much more effective than any of these.

Benzoyl Peroxide—Often Effective for Mild Cases of Acne

Ironically, the newest innovation in the over-the-counter treatment of acne was first used in medicine in 1920. Benzoyl peroxide was found to be effective for acne in the mid-1970s and since then has become the most reliable OTC treatment for mild cases of acne.

Benzoyl peroxide, the active ingredient in products like Benoxyl lotion and Oxy-5 and Oxy-10, has several desirable effects on acne. It kills bacteria that contribute to the inflammatory process, it removes some of the excess oil, and most importantly, it prevents sebum from getting clogged inside skin pores.

Unfortunately, benzoyl peroxide can also mess up your skin if you don't use it properly. The drug is a skin irritant, and you have to allow yourself an opportunity to work up to its full effects.

People with sensitive skin should start with a 5 percent concentration of the drug—for instance, Oxy-5. After washing with a mild soap and water, gently rub a small amount of medication into the skin. Be sure not to get any in your eyes, mouth, nose, or on your lips. Let the drug sit on your skin for about fifteen minutes, then wash it off.

Repeat this procedure each night for a week, increasing your contact time by fifteen minutes per night. At the end of a week your skin should be able to tolerate the drug overnight. Be sure to wash it all off the next morning.

Up to 10 percent of people find that benzoyl peroxide is too irritating and have to stop using it. The drug may cause reddening and drying of the skin or even swelling in treated areas. Reactions are more common in people with fair, sensitive skin. They are also more likely to occur in people who spend much time in the sun. Don't try to get a tan if you are using benzoyl peroxide.

It's common to feel a mild burning sensation when you start using benzoyl peroxide. You will probably also experience skin peeling during the first month of treatment. Most side effects can be handled by temporarily decreasing exposure time or by discontinuing treatments for a few days.

Be especially careful about applying benzoyl peroxide to your neck. The skin there seems to be particularly sensitive to the irritant effects of the drug. You should also avoid getting this stuff on your clothes, bed sheets, eyebrows, and hair. Benzoyl peroxide is chemically related to the hydrogen peroxide that bleaches hair and clothing. If you aren't careful, you could end up with speckled hair and ruined clothes.

Blacks experience a unique problem with this drug. Since benzoyl peroxide causes mild skin peeling, they look as if they have a dirty ash on their faces. Many blacks understandably find this cosmetically intolerable.

If your skin tolerates 5 percent benzoyl peroxide gels or lotions well, you can move up to one of the 10 percent products. But be careful. You need to repeat the slow buildup procedure when you go to a higher strength.

Don't self-medicate with benzoyl peroxide or any other acne product if you are seeing a doctor for your acne. Benzoyl peroxide can complicate other treatments and can seriously injure your skin if your doctor doesn't know you are using it in combination with prescription drugs.

Soaps and Cleansers—Potential for Damage

Beauty may be skin deep, but acne has deeper roots.

Acne develops below the surface of the skin, where no soap or cleanser can reach. Since there's no way you can clean out the inside of a clogged follicle, you can't get at the source of the problem with a soap. The most you can hope to accomplish is to clear excess oil off the surface of the skin. And any soap should be able to do that; you don't need high-powered anti-acne abrasive cleansers and scrubs.

Studies have shown that some of the abrasives may actually do more harm than good. Abrasives, which scratch away the outermost layer of skin, may reduce the numbers of pimples on your face for a few weeks, but some people end up with more pimples a couple of months later than they had when they started.

A mild soap applied with a soft washcloth is probably all you need. If your skin is exceptionally oily, you may need to wash your face during the day. Cleansing pads containing alcohol, acetone, or mild soap are easier to carry than regular soap. These products do a good job and may speed up acne healing.

Soaps may also contain old drugs like resorcinol, salicylic acid, and sulfur. While these relics of a bygone era may have some benefit in acne lotions and creams, they are practically useless in soaps. Any drug for acne has to sit on the surface of the skin long enough to soak into the inflamed follicles. When you use a soap, how long do you let it stay on your skin? Usually less than a minute—then you wash it off. When you wash off a ''medicated'' soap, the medication goes down the drain with the soap.

Save yourself some money and forget about special acne soaps.

᠊᠊᠊᠊᠊᠊᠊᠊᠊᠊᠊᠊᠊᠊

The Pharmacist's Prescription for Acne

General Information
OTC treatment only controls acne, it doesn't cure it. Do what you can to limit outbreaks.

Recommended Treatment
Keep your skin clean, but don't wash more than three times a day.

Wash with a mild soap, massage your skin gently with a soft cloth, and pat dry with a soft towel.

Avoid any products that irritate your skin, including colognes and aftershaves with high alcohol content.

Don't pick at your pimples. That just makes them come back worse the next time.

Avoid greasy or oily cosmetics.

Try a benzoyl peroxide product and follow the directions given earlier in this chapter.

See the Doctor if . . .
- Your self-treatment is not effective or makes your acne worse.
- You have hard lumps, or cysts, under your skin.
- You have inflamed patches over large areas of your face or body.
- You are over twenty years of age.

Products Recommended for Acne
Cleansers
Betadine Skin Cleanser
Noxzema Antiseptic Skin Cleanser
Seba-Nil

Benzoyl peroxide
Benoxyl Lotion   Clearasil Benzoyl Peroxide
                                  Lotion

Clearasil BP Acne
  Treatment
Cuticura Acne Cream
Fostex Gel

Loroxide Lotion
Oxy-5
Oxy-10
Oxy Wash
Vanoxide Lotion

Or the generic equivalent of any of the above

Products Not Recommended for Self-Medication of Acne

Acne-Aid (B)
Acnomel (B)
Clearasil Acne
  Treatment Stick (B)
Clearasil Antibacterial
  Soap (C)
Clearasil Pore Deep
  Cleanser (B)
Cuticura Medicated
  Soap (C)
Cuticura Ointment (B)
Fostex Soap (C)
Fostril Lotion (B)

Komed Lotion (B)
Komex Cleanser (B)
Liquimat Lotion (B)
Medicated Face
  Conditioner (B)
Multiscrub (B)
Pernox Lotion (B)
pHisoAc (B)
pHisoDerm Cleanser (B)
Rezamid Lotion (B)
Stri-Dex Medicated
  Pads (B)
Sulfur Soap (C)

Or the generic equivalent of any of the above

The products listed in the "Not Recommended" tables are not recommended by me for one or more of the following reasons: (A) One or more ingredients have been reported to be ineffective or only slightly effective for the product's intended purpose; (B) a more effective product is available; (C) the product advertising or description is likely to heighten consumer expectation beyond actual effectiveness; (D) the product has the potential to cause side effects in the average consumer that are more serious than those generally associated with OTC drugs; (E) the product has the potential to cause serious side effects in persons with specific diseases or disorders; (F) another product is available that is capable of producing the same or nearly the same therapeutic effect without the same risk of side effects; (G) persistent use of the product may cause physical dependency that alters an otherwise normal body function; (H) the product's formulation may reduce the effectiveness of one of its ingredients; (I) this is a multiple-ingredient product that may have no therapeutic advantage over simpler or single-ingredient products; (J) one or more of the product's ingredients may be useful for only a short period during the total duration of the illness; (K) the product cannot easily be administered at a dosage level within generally recommended boundaries of optimal therapeutic effect; (L) this is a condition-specific product that is appropriate for use only after a health professional has helped the patient establish a diagnosis.

Sunburn—A Common Cause of Skin Damage

Sunburn is the most common type of burn. While severe sunburn can be dangerous, even lethal, most sunburns are only nuisances. Most sunburns can be self-treated, but any sunburn that produces watery blisters under the skin, becomes infected, or makes you physically ill should be treated by a doctor.

The sun affects different people to different degrees. Anyone who spends enough time in the sun will burn, but some are much more sensitive than others.

Your degree of sun sensitivity depends primarily on your skin type and, oddly enough, on the color of your eyes and hair.

Some people are genetically predetermined to be sensitive to the burning rays of the sun. Those with fair skin, freckles, red hair, and green or hazel eyes are most sensitive. These folks should avoid the sun whenever possible and should wear a sunscreen and protective clothing when they have to be in the sun.

Blacks are at the other extreme. They can have fun in the sun with relative impunity. It is much harder for them to burn than it is for those of northern European descent. Native Americans, Asian Indians, Orientals, and people of Mediterranean descent occupy an intermediate position.

Nobody wants a sunburn—what we want is a healthy-looking tan. What's the difference and how does the sun affect your skin?

A burn is your skin's reaction to excess energy. As far as the skin is concerned, it doesn't matter if you lie on a blanket on the beach all day or throw a bucket of scalding water on yourself. The immediate result is the same. The important difference, however, is that the sun (or a sunlamp) produces radiation damage. This has long-term effects that accumulate over a lifetime.

Sunburn is a burn, but it takes longer for the skin to redden after sun exposure than with other burns. In fact, it takes twelve to twenty-four hours for maximal lobstering.

What's so bad about light? Aren't we exposed to it all day and most of the night? Why should the sun cause such a problem?

The light that the sun emits isn't a problem at all—it's the radiation that comes with it. Any time, whether summer or winter, that we step out into sunlight, we are exposed to ultraviolet radiation. And that's the cause of sunburn.

Actually, most of the ultraviolet (UV) radiation that the sun beams toward earth is absorbed by the ozone layer in the atmosphere above us. But we still have problems with the radiation that gets through that protective envelope.

Ultraviolet radiation is present in three energy levels, UV-A, UV-B, and UV-C. UV-C is the least troublesome because the ozone layer manages to absorb almost all of it. Of the two remaining energy levels, UV-B is the more dangerous. UV-B can cause severe sunburn with blistering, fever, chills, and weakness.

UV-A, the so-called tanning ray, is thought to be less dangerous but can still cause sunburn, especially in light-complexioned people. While UV-A radiation may be "safer" than the other two energy levels, there is no safe form of UV radiation.

What's so bad about a little sunburn? Won't you eventually tan and then be able to tolerate more sun the next time?

A good tan is attractive. Well-tanned people catch a second glance when they pass by. But what's the cost of a good cosmetic appearance?

A tan is a sign of skin damage. The deeper the tan, the more your skin has been insulted and the greater the likelihood of future skin problems. Your skin has the memory of an elephant. You can't abuse it year after year without paying the price. And that price may be stiff.

The most serious effect of chronic tanning is skin cancer. This year 400,000 *new* cases of skin cancer will be treated. That doesn't include the number of precancerous lesions that will be treated or the cases of skin cancer that will be retreated!

Signs of Skin Cancer

A mole that changes colors
A birthmark or skin blemish that changes colors
A sore or red mark on the skin that does not go away
A bump on the skin that does not go away or gets larger
A patch of skin that bleeds easily

The box above lists some of the common signs of skin cancer. If any of these apply to you, get yourself to the doctor as soon as you can. The most common types of skin cancer are basal cell carcinoma, squamous cell carcinoma, and malignant melanoma. The first two are easily treated in the doctor's office. In fact, the cancer on President Reagan's nose was a basal cell.

The third type of skin cancer, malignant melanoma, is a different story. This form can rapidly invade the tissues under the skin, release malignant cells into the blood, and attack other areas of the body. Malignant melanoma is rapidly fatal if left untreated but can be controlled if diagnosed early.

In short, don't take chances with skin problems. Get them checked out early and then feel confident that you have nothing to worry about.

Who is at greatest risk of skin cancer? The same groups who have the most trouble with sunburn, plus people like construction workers and farmers, whose jobs require that they work long hours in the sun. A redheaded, freckled farmer, for instance, should take extra precautions to avoid sun exposure.

But skin cancer isn't the only or even the most common problem associated with long-term sun exposure. The constant cycle of sun exposure, skin damage, tanning reaction, and more sun exposure leads to permanent deterioration of the elastic structures of the skin. This destruction produces a dark, leathery, yellow, wrinkled skin. These changes are almost identical to those seen with natural aging.

As if this weren't enough, the skin becomes dry and cracked, may develop spiderlike blood vessels on the surface, skin growths, and bleeding in the lower layers of the skin. As the process continues, the skin becomes thinner and is more easily damaged by the sun, abrasions, insect bites, and any other skin irritant.

We've all seen people who look ten to fifteen years older than their actual age just because they decided to roast themselves at the beach or pool every summer. And all of this is in the name of beauty! And now, thanks to tanning booths, we can fry our skin all year round.

Dermatologists tell us that *there is no such thing as a safe tanning booth.* We should heed their warnings. Tanning spa operators are quick to point out that their booths are safer than the sun, that more than 95 percent of their radiation (although they avoid using that word) is in the form of UV-A, and that they filter out almost all skin burning UV-B radiation.

But what effect does UV-A radiation have on the skin?

UV-A is less likely to produce sunburn than are the other forms of ultraviolet radiation, but UV-A penetrates deep into the skin and damages the small blood vessels that supply the skin. Tanning booths don't protect you from premature skin aging.

What are the long-term effects of tanning booths? Only time will tell. Tanning spas are a relatively new phenomenon. It will take several years to establish either their safety or the degree of damage that they cause. Just consider that in terms of the energy your skin soaks up, lying in a tanning bed is little different than baking your flesh in an oven.

Preventing Sunburn

Fortunately, many people are paying attention to the warnings about sun exposure. By 1990, suntan and sunscreen products will reach almost a half billion dollars in annual sales. In terms of sales volume, this makes them the largest class of dermatologic products. Unfortunately, the megabucks that are involved also draw advertising that makes the use and selection of sunscreens much more complicated than they need to be.

In many cases, you don't need to use a sunscreen if you take proper precautions when you're in the sun. Even if you don't mind smearing up with a gooey lotion, there will be times when you'll be caught without it.

In most of the United States, the rays of the sun are most direct and damaging between 10:00 A.M. and 2:00 P.M. It's best to limit your sun exposure during these hours. Clouds offer no protection at all. Clouds are simply water vapor and are incapable of blocking any ultraviolet radiation. Some of the worst sunburns I've ever seen happened on cloudy days. Likewise, water in a swimming pool lets almost all the UV rays pass through to the swimmer. The little bit of energy that doesn't get through is reflected off the surface and bakes your chin and neck.

What about sitting under an umbrella at the beach? It's better than nothing, but sand is a good energy reflector. Its reflections can cook you under your umbrella, where you least expect it.

Do things get better in winter? A little, but not much. The sun's rays aren't as direct in winter, and you probably won't be outside as much as in summer. But be careful if you plan to go skiing. Snow reflects almost 100 percent of the UV radiation that hits it. Unprepared skiers usually return home with serious sunburns on their faces and necks.

Okay, so those are some of the things we should not do. What are some things that work?

Clothing—The Best Protection

If you are aware of radiation reflectors, like sand, snow, and water, you can plan some protection for yourself. Clothing is the best sun protector. When practical, wear a cap or hat, polarized sunglasses, and cover as much skin as you can with clothing. T-shirts are better than tank tops, but long sleeves are better yet. Shorts are better than a skimpy swimsuit, but long pants or jeans are more protective.

If you wear a shirt for protection at poolside, make sure it stays dry. Dry clothes block practically all UV rays, but wet clothes allow as much as 50 percent of the radiation to pass through to the skin.

Sunscreens—Burn Reduction, Not Prevention

If you don't want to look peculiar at poolside or risk overheating in the summer, you can use a sunscreen. Sunscreens basically do what their name implies; they screen out the sun. They protect exposed areas of skin from burning, prevent premature aging, and, we hope, reduce the chances of skin cancer.

The FDA has approved three basic types of sunscreens.

1. Sunscreen-sunburn preventive agents, which absorb 95 percent of the sun's UV radiation
2. Sunscreen-suntan agents, which absorb only 85 percent of the sun's rays
3. Sunscreen-opaque agents, which reflect virtually all UV radiation (but these agents are white pastes that are cosmetically appropriate only for lifeguards' noses)

The thick pastes like zinc oxide and titanium dioxide ointments obviously work by physically shielding the skin from the sun. The other sunscreens, like para-aminobenzoic acid (PABA), actually absorb UV radiation before it can interact with the skin.

There are more than twenty chemically distinct sunscreen ingredients on the market, but PABA is the most common and probably the most effective. No single sunscreen is capable of blocking all wavelengths of UV radiation. Therefore, sunscreens are one of the few examples of over-the-counter drugs where combinations are preferable to single-agent products.

Rather than judging by a product's ingredients, it is generally more helpful to select a product based on its Sun Protection Factor, or SPF. Products currently on the market have SPF's ranging from 2 to 23. The number indicates the comparative amount of time it takes to produce sunburn.

For instance, if you know that you normally start to burn after a ten-minute sun exposure, a product with an SPF of 10 will let you stay out ten times that long, or 100 minutes. A sunscreen with an SPF value of 15 would allow you to stay in the sun for 10×15 (150) minutes.

The important thing to remember is that *sunscreens only reduce burning,* they don't altogether prevent it.

There are elaborate charts that can help you select a sunscreen based on your skin type and eye color, but I don't recommend them. Since the only good sun exposure is no exposure, I suggest that you stick to products with an SPF of 15.

One exception to this advice pertains to small children. Infants can absorb the ingredients of the sunscreen through the skin. Consequently, children less than six months old should not be given sunscreens with an SPF of greater than 4. It is best to ask your pediatrician or dermatologist about the proper sunscreen for children from infancy to teens.

If you use a sunscreen, be sure to use it correctly. These products work best if they are applied at least thirty minutes before going out in the sun. This allows the chemical time to soak into your skin and work most effectively.

Water is a natural enemy of sunscreens. Even so-called "water-proof" products can still wash off after ninety minutes of swimming. Try to reapply the cream or lotion frequently if you are sweating heavily or swimming.

Like every other drug, sunscreens can cause side effects. These are usually rashes that are caused either by a direct irritating effect on the skin or by allergy. If this happens to you, let your pharmacist help you select another product with different ingredients.

Tanning Lotions—Some Good Choices, Some Bad Choices

Ironically, the better tanning lotions don't produce suntans; they suppress them. Most of them contain sunscreens that slow burning and thus slow the skin's response—the tan. They also lubricate the skin, trapping its natural moisture to minimize harmful dehydrating effects of the sun.

Some people prefer to use homemade tanning lotions. They apply baby oil (which is nothing more than perfumed mineral oil), iodine in oil, or cocoa butter. Baby oil and cocoa butter provide no protection from the sun. Baby oil not only lets all the sun's ultraviolet radiation pass through to the skin, but also traps body heat in the skin. Baby oil fries your skin like chicken in a skillet. Cocoa butter does about the same thing.

Why use iodine in baby oil? Iodine's brownish color darkens a natural tan and enhances the effect. Dyes have been used in commercial suntan lotions for years, and the practice doesn't make any more sense than using iodine. The enhanced tans from dyes and iodine don't look natural. If you don't wash the stuff off your hands, your palms become darker than the rest of your skin. And that really looks peculiar.

A synthetic dye called canthaxanthin is now being used in tablet or capsule form as an oral tanning agent. Supposedly you can take several doses of this and tan without even going out in the sun.

When canthaxanthin works, it discolors the fat cells underneath the skin, giving the skin surface a tanned appearance. However, its manufacturer is not required by the FDA to submit any information about its safety because the chemical is legally considered a food dye and not a drug.

The bottom line on canthaxanthin and any other oral "tanning" agent is to stay away from it until somebody proves that it is both safe and effective.

Treating a Sunburn

No matter how many precautions you may take, sunburn is inevitable sometime during the summer. What should you do after the burn?

The overall objectives in treating a sunburn are to relieve pain and to promote healing. While these are laudable objectives, no product on the market does a good job in either situation.

One of the best things you can do for a sunburn is to keep the skin moist. Emollient creams like Nivea, Nutraplus, Nutraderm, and Eucerin trap moisture inside the skin. In so doing, they reduce blistering and peeling and minimize the tight feeling the skin gets after a burn.

Nothing speeds the healing of a sunburn. Nothing reduces the damage that the sun has already done. Tincture of time is the only proven cure for sunburn. Burns need to heal naturally. Therefore, we have to be careful about what we slap on the skin. We have to be sure that our "treatment" doesn't actually prolong the problem.

Local Anesthetics—For Short-term Relief Only

Some say that local anesthetics impede rather than promote healing. At first glance local anesthetics—for example, benzocaine—drugs that wipe out pain sensations in the skin, appear to be the ideal treatment for the pain of a sunburn. The problem is that most of these preparations have difficulty crossing through the top layer of skin to get to the underlying nerves. Anesthetics have to act on nerves, not on skin cells.

The first problem with local anesthetics, particularly benzocaine, is that no one is sure of the effective dose. One study of benzocaine has demonstrated that you need to apply a 20 percent concentration of the drug to the skin to achieve any pain relief for normal or mildly burned skin. Other studies have shown that concentrations as low as 5 percent may be effective for severe burns. Very few products contain 20 percent benzocaine; Americaine is one example, but several have less than 5 percent, including Foille and Unguentine aerosol sprays.

The second problem with anesthetics is that they may sensitize the skin to allergic reactions. One out of every hundred people who use benzocaine on their skin develops an allergic rash from it. Even though the percentages are in your favor, if you are that one person, an allergic reaction on top of a sunburn is guaranteed to be a painful mess.

Local anesthetics have even more limitations. They don't work for very long and you must restrict the amount you use each day. The anesthetics' action lasts for only thirty to forty-five minutes. In other words, an hour after you apply your medication, you'll want to use some more.

Don't do it.

The anesthetic that passes through the layers of skin eventually gets into your blood and finds its way to your heart and central nervous system. Overdoses of local anesthetics can irritate your nerves and alter your heartbeat.

Don't apply local anesthetics more often than four times a day, and don't apply them to large areas of the body, because in doing so you increase your body's exposure to them. Badly damaged skin allows more anesthetic to pass into the blood than does normal, intact skin. Therefore, don't apply local anesthetics to raw, blistered, or badly burned skin.

Curiously, antihistamines applied directly to the skin are also fairly good local anesthetics. The best known of these is Caladryl lotion, a combination of calamine lotion and the antihistamine Benadryl. But they have the same limitations as the drugs we generally think of as anesthetics. They don't work well on intact skin, and they can cause allergic reactions.

Astringents—For a Cooling Effect

Astringents are agents that reduce swelling from sunburn. Calamine lotion is the best known of these. As the lotion dries on the skin the evaporation process cools the skin and gives some temporary relief.

An even better remedy is Burow's solution. This is commercially available as Domeboro tablets or powder. Follow the directions on the container to make a solution from the tablets or powder. This medication is for external use only; *do not take Domeboro by mouth*. To apply, dip a clean cotton cloth in the solution, wring it out, and place the cloth over the burn. Repeat the procedure as often as you wish. The solution has a cooling effect on the skin and also keeps it moist.

Anti-Inflammatory Drugs—Better Aspirin Than Hydrocortisone

The anti-inflammatory hydrocortisone products that are currently available over the counter are probably too weak to be of much help in sunburn. Even the potent hydrocortisone derivatives your doctor can prescribe have only limited benefit in sunburn. Sometimes oral doses of these drugs can relieve severe cases of sunburn, but they are only available by prescription.

But there is one OTC anti-inflammatory drug that may be of benefit—aspirin. Normal doses of aspirin seem to alter the body's response to sunburn. While I wouldn't expect the burn to go away any faster with aspirin, you may find that it relieves some of the pain and inflammation. Be sure to read the dosing information and precautions concerning aspirin in chapter 3. If you can't take aspirin, acetaminophen (e.g., Datril, Tylenol) or ibuprofen (e.g., Advil, Nuprin) may give you some relief.

The Pharmacist's Prescription for Sunburn

General Information
Prevention is the best treatment. Limit your sun exposure, wear protective clothing, including a hat that shades your face, and use a sunscreen when you have to be out in the sun.

Recommended Treatment
Apply a mild astringent like calamine lotion or Burow's solution.

Local anesthetics can give a few minutes of relief. Don't use them more than four times a day, and don't apply them over large areas or to blistered or broken skin.

Aerosols are easier and less painful to apply than creams and lotions.

Aspirin or acetaminophen may relieve some of the burn pain.

See the Doctor if . . .
• Your sunburn was caused by a sunlamp.
• You develop a fever.
• Your skin starts to swell or to develop watery blisters.
• You feel that you have no energy.
• You develop a skin infection.

Products Recommended for Treatment of Sunburn

Local anesthetics
  Americaine Aerosol
  Lanacane Lotion

Analgesics (to be taken by mouth)
  Acetaminophen
  Aspirin
  Ibuprofen

Astringents
  Calamine Lotion
  Domeboro
    Or the generic equivalent of any of the above

Products Not Recommended for Self-Medication of Sunburn

Dermoplast (l)   Solarcaine(l)

Foille (k)   Unguentine (K,l)

Or the generic equivalent of any of the above

The products listed in the "Not Recommended" tables are not recommended by me for one or more of the following reasons: (A) One or more ingredients have been reported to be ineffective or only slightly effective for the product's intended purpose; (B) a more effective product is available; (C) the product advertising or description is likely to heighten consumer expectation beyond actual effectiveness; (D) the product has the potential to cause side effects in the average consumer that are more serious than those generally associated with OTC drugs; (E) the product has the potential to cause serious side effects in persons with specific diseases or disorders; (F) another product is available that is capable of producing the same or nearly the same therapeutic effect without the same risk of side effects; (G) persistent use of the product may cause physical dependency that alters an otherwise normal body function; (H) the product's formulation may reduce the effectiveness of one of its ingredients; (I) this is a multiple-ingredient product that may have no therapeutic advantage over simpler or single-ingredient products; (J) one or more of the product's ingredients may be useful for only a short period during the total duration of the illness; (K) the product cannot easily be administered at a dosage level within generally recommended boundaries of optimal therapeutic effect; (L) this is a condition-specific product that is appropriate for use only after a health professional has helped the patient establish a diagnosis.

Age Spots and Other Skin Discolorations

Everyone's skin gets discolored with age, and there's nothing to worry about, right?

Wrong!

Aging does cause some people to develop dark splotches on their skin, but not all skin discolorations are harmless. In some cases, they may appear with glandular diseases, liver problems, pregnancy, skin cancer, and even with the use of drugs such as tranquilizers, estrogens, and oral contraceptives.

Since skin discolorations may be signs of serious medical problems, they should be checked by a doctor. Fortunately, the most common skin discolorations are benign, and these include freckles, melasma, and age spots.

Freckles are simply collections of the pigment melanin,

which gives the skin a speckled appearance. Melasma, the mask of pregnancy, is caused by hormone-related melanin deposits in the skin. Age spots, more properly called solar or senile lentigines, are also masses of melanin and appear primarily on the face, hands, and arms.

Each of these conditions has two characteristics in common with the others: They are all caused by deposits of melanin near the surface of the skin, and they are all made worse by exposure to the sun.

If freckles, melasma, or age spots are a problem for you, stay out of the sun. If you can't do that, at least wear protective clothing and a sunscreen. (See the section earlier in this chapter on prevention of sunburn.)

But what about the pigment itself? Can you do anything about that?

Yes, to some extent.

Skin Lighteners—Partially Effective for Some

You can use products known as "skin bleaches" to help lighten the color of the melanin pigments in your skin. But don't expect them to go away completely.

The only skin bleach or skin lightener approved by the FDA advisory panel is hydroquinolone, the ingredient found in Eldoquin, Esoterica, and Porcelana. This drug is intended to disrupt the function of melanin in the skin and to lighten the blotches it causes.

How effective is hydroquinolone? That depends upon what you expect it to do.

Hydroquinolone is more effective for people with lighter skin color and lighter spots. In other words, it doesn't work as well for those who need it most.

Eldoquin, Esoterica, and Porcelana each contain a 2 percent concentration of hydroquinolone. This strength is generally considered safe, although some people experience burning and skin inflammation when they apply it. It also irritates the eyes if it accidentally gets there.

These creams or lotions should be gently rubbed into affected areas twice a day. But don't expect anything to happen overnight. It usually takes several weeks to achieve maximal effect. If you don't see any change within two months, you might as well give up and see whether your dermatologist can help you.

If you're one of the lucky ones who achieves the effect you want, you'll need to continue regular use. You may be able to cut down to one application a day, or even every other day, but the pigmentation will slowly return if you completely stop using the medication.

But what about those who don't get the results they had hoped for?

They have three choices: (1) They can be satisfied with a partial improvement and maintain that; (2) they can give up and learn to accept their skin pigmentation; or (3) they can up the ante.

The first two choices are viable alternatives, but I don't recommend the last. The FDA advisory panel found that hydroquinolone concentrations of 4 percent or more caused an unacceptable risk of side effects. Not only can this drug cause skin inflammation, but in high doses it can cause the skin to thicken and even turn yellow!

If you decide to use one of these products, be sure to use it as the manufacturer intended. Read and follow all directions carefully. Stop using it if it irritates your skin or if you don't see any improvement within two months.

Poison Ivy

Poison ivy rash is a form of contact dermatitis, a rash caused by physical contact with an allergen. In this case it's caused by a plant. While poison ivy, poison oak, and poison sumac are distinctly different plants, the reactions they cause are almost identical. In terms of OTC treatment, it doesn't matter whether one of these or one of the sixty other plants that commonly cause contact dermatitis is the root of the problem. They're all treated the same way.

The Symptoms of Poison Ivy

For simplicity's sake, we'll refer to all of these weed rashes as ''poison ivy.'' It usually takes the rash two to three days to develop after exposure. The delay between exposure and the appearance of the rash may make it difficult to determine where and when the contact was made.

After the incubation period, a red, weeping rash develops in all the areas exposed to a resin in the plant's sap. The rashes often look like red streaks across the skin, since most people brush against the plants as they walk through wooded areas.

Poison ivy rashes feel hot, swollen, and itchy. Most form small, liquid blisters under the skin. As the lesions begin to heal, these blisters either dissolve into the skin or break, leaving crusts on the skin surface. Broken blisters are susceptible to bacterial infections, the most common complication of poison ivy.

Most cases of poison ivy are mild and self-limited. They go away in two to three weeks without treatment. But those two to three weeks are miserable!

Myths and Misconceptions About Poison Ivy

Washing Poison Ivy Away—Only if You Hurry

Many people believe that they can come home from a day in the woods, bathe with a strong soap or detergent, and prevent weed rashes.

Close, but not quite right.

You can wash poison ivy resin off your skin, but washing does no good unless you do it *within ten minutes* of exposure. That's how long it takes for the allergen to get down into your skin and start the allergic reaction.

Bathing after a hike or picnic in the weeds may wash off dirt and bugs, but not poison ivy.

Spreading Poison Ivy to Others—You Can't

Poison ivy is not contagious. You can't spread it to your friends or family. You can't even spread it from one part of your own body to another.

But it sure looks as if the stuff marches up and down your arms and legs, doesn't it? Appearances are deceiving. Since the rash takes several days to incubate, more sensitive or more heavily exposed areas of skin react first. Hours or even days later, other patches of skin take their turn at erupting. This gives the false impression that the rash is moving and engulfing healthy skin. In fact, only skin that is directly exposed to the plant's resin reacts. And you can't give poison ivy to anyone else. They have to come into direct contact with the toxic resin.

Getting Poison Ivy Long Distance—Contact Is Required

Some people claim to get poison ivy rashes if they just look at a plant. Not true. Poison ivy is a stationary plant; it can't jump out at you. What usually happens to these people is that they become exposed without realizing it.

A chemical, urushiol, found in the plant's resin is responsible for the allergic reaction. We come into contact with this resin when we injure the plant. I wouldn't advise it, but most people can carefully pick up and handle intact poison ivy plants without getting a rash. But if you tear or scrape a leaf or stem, you'll get some of the resin on you and will probably develop a rash.

The only ways you can get poison ivy are to touch an injured plant, to become exposed to resin-filled smoke from burning plants, or to come into contact with urushiol from other sources.

What are these other sources?

You can't spread poison ivy from your rash to another person, but you can spread the resin. For instance, you can catch poison ivy from resin deposits on your child's clothes or shoes. You can even get it from petting a dog or cat that has been in the woods.

Most people who claim to get poison ivy by long distance actually make contact with it from these types of secondary exposures.

Preventing Poison Ivy Rashes

There is no sure way to prevent poison ivy. Even if you stay away from wooded areas, you can still get it from your garden, from your kids' clothes, or from Fido.

Clothing is the best prevention if you know you will be going into an area where poison ivy exposure is likely. Dress so that as much skin is covered as possible. Wear a long-sleeved shirt, long pants, shoes, and socks. Thin cotton gloves may also help. When you return from the area where the plant grows, make sure you wash all these items carefully (including your shoes). Be careful to avoid exposing your skin to any resin that may be lurking on the clothes.

Some dermatologists and allergists can desensitize highly susceptible people with poison ivy extract injections. This is a long process that may only make reactions less severe. A few poison ivy "vaccines" are available over the counter, but they aren't extremely effective either. Nor are they free of side effects like stomach upset and rectal itching.

If poison ivy is a serious problem for you, see your doctor. Don't mess around with OTC poison ivy vaccines.

Treating Poison Ivy

Comfort yourself with the thought that poison ivy is self-limited; it will go away on its own. Don't do anything that will complicate matters. Don't insist on self-treatments if your rash is small or healing nicely. On the other hand, waste no time in getting to the doctor if you know you are extremely sensitive to poison ivy or if large areas of your body are involved.

While most cases of poison ivy are mild and uncomplicated, the itching can be maddening. OTC products for poison ivy are similar to those for sunburn, but one basic rule of dermatology especially applies to poison ivy: If the rash is wet, dry it; if the rash is dry, wet it.

In the early stages, poison ivy rashes are wet and weeping. These should be "dried" with products like the astringents listed below. Never put an ointment on a weeping rash; it will make a disgusting mess.

On the other hand, if the rash dries out in its last days, it is more responsive to ointment forms of the anesthetics and anti-inflammatory drugs listed below.

Astringents—Some Temporary Relief

Astringents like calamine or Burow's solution may give some temporary relief, but don't expect too much from them.

The main problem with calamine for poison ivy is that it dries, leaving a powdery crust that is difficult and painful to remove. Bacteria can set up shop in this crust, and a serious skin infection can result. I don't recommend calamine lotion for poison ivy unless I can monitor the patient closely. Burow's solution is much less of a problem. This preparation can give significant relief and can be applied several times a day. See the section on sunburn earlier earlier in this chapter for directions.

Antiseptics—Little Practical Value

Antiseptics in poison ivy products have more theoretical than practical value. These drugs are supposed to suppress the bacteria on the skin, thus preventing infections. Unfortunately, their effectiveness for this purpose has not been clearly established.

Antipruritics—Some Relief, Some Risk

The two major groups of antipruritic, or anti-itch, drugs are the same local anesthetics discussed in the section on sunburns and the counter-irritants.

The local anesthetics have the same benefits and liabilities as those mentioned in the previous section. In fact, they are the very same drugs. They can provide relief for up to an hour, but they also carry the risk of allergic reactions.

Some people get good relief from counter-irritants like menthol and camphor, but I have reservations about recommending an irritant for inflamed skin. The theory behind these agents is described in chapter 3. They basically work by irritating the skin, confusing the nerves inside the skin and causing a paradoxical cooling sensation on the surface of the skin.

Anti-Inflammatory Drugs—Marginally Effective

Hydrocortisone is the most effective OTC drug for treatment of poison ivy rash, but that isn't saying much. Hydrocortisone reduces some of the inflammation of a poison ivy rash, but it still takes a couple of days for it to reduce itching sensations.

The FDA limits OTC concentrations of hydrocortisone to 0.5 percent, which is only marginally effective. The drug also has one unique and potentially hazardous side effect—it can spread infections.

Corticosteroid drugs, the class that includes hydrocortisone, are well known for their anti-inflammatory effects.

They reduce inflammation by suppressing the body's immune system. Unfortunately, the immune suppression also allows bacteria to grow faster.

Other, more potent corticosteroids are available by prescription. If you aren't making satisfactory progress with your poison ivy, go see the doctor. The visit may be well worth it. Don't put too much faith or invest too much time in OTC treatments.

Antihistamines—Relief by Sedation?

If poison ivy is an allergic reaction, taking an antihistamine should be just the ticket, right?

Oral doses of antihistamines can be beneficial in treating poison ivy, but not for the apparent reason. Taking an antihistamine to diminish a poison ivy rash is like closing the barn door after the horse has escaped. Antihistamines are much more effective if they are taken *before* exposure to an allergen.

But antihistamines do give some relief. Many dermatologists recommend them because they cause drowsiness as a side effect, and they have found that their patients itch and scratch less if they are sedated. Of course, sedation can cause other problems. Sedation can make it more difficult to concentrate on your work, can make driving a car more dangerous, and can pose physical hazards if you have to operate dangerous machinery while you take the drug.

Any of the OTC antihistamines can cause drowsiness, but diphenhydramine (brand name Benadryl) is more sedating than the others. (You can find a more complete listing and description of the actions and side effects of the antihistamines in chapter 2.)

The Pharmacist's Prescription for Poison Ivy

General Information

Prevent or limit the effects of poison ivy by dressing properly before exposure. Launder clothing carefully after returning from a potential exposure.

Treatment may provide some relief from inflammation and

itching. Lasting relief generally depends on subsidence of the allergic reaction over time.

Recommended Treatment

Apply hydrocortisone lotion or cream up to four times a day to poison ivy lesions unless infection is present.

Use Burow's solution soaks for temporary relief of itching and burning.

Use an antihistamine to reduce itching sensations.

See the Doctor if . . .

- You can't control your itching and scratching.
- Your rash involves a large area of your body.
- You have poison ivy close to your eyes.
- You have large blisters developing.
- Your blisters exude a yellowish material.
- Your skin or the underlying tissue begins to swell.
- You have a fever.

Products Recommended for Poison Ivy

Astringents
Calamine Lotion
Domeboro

Anesthetics
Americaine Spray
Lanacane Lotion

Anti-inflammatory agents
Caldecort Cream
Clinicort Cream
Cortaid Cream
Dermolate Cream
Lanacort Cream

Antihistamine
Benadryl
Or the generic equivalent of any of the above

Products Not Recommended for Self-Medication of Poison Ivy

Caladryl (I)
Ivarest (I)
Ivy Dry Cream (I)
Ivy-Rid (B)
Rhuli Cream (I,K)

Rhuli Spray (I,K)
Rhuligel (I)
Rhulihist (I,K)
Ziradryl (I)

Or the generic equivalent of any of the above

The products listed in the "Not Recommended" tables are not recommended by me for one or more of the following reasons: (A) One or more ingredients have been reported to be ineffective or only slightly effective for the product's intended purpose; (B) a more effective product is available; (C) the product advertising or description is likely to heighten consumer expectation beyond actual effectiveness; (D) the product has the potential to cause side effects in the average consumer that are more serious than those generally associated with OTC drugs; (E) the product has the potential to cause serious side effects in persons with specific diseases or disorders; (F) another product is available that is capable of producing the same or nearly the same therapeutic effect without the same risk of side effects; (G) persistent use of the product may cause physical dependency that alters an otherwise normal body function; (H) the product's formulation may reduce the effectiveness of one of its ingredients; (I) this is a multiple-ingredient product that may have no therapeutic advantage over simpler or single-ingredient products; (J) one or more of the product's ingredients may be useful for only a short period during the total duration of the illness; (K) the product cannot easily be administered at a dosage level within generally recommended boundaries of optimal therapeutic effect; (L) this is a condition-specific product that is appropriate for use only after a health professional has helped the patient establish a diagnosis.

Bacterial Skin Infections

One of the things the skin does best is defend itself and the rest of the body from bacteria. Many of the infections that occur on skin originate from bacteria that find their way into hair follicles or sweat glands. These infections can develop into boils and carbuncles.

Damage to the surface of the skin can lead to superficial infections like impetigo. These infections can get their start from cuts and scrapes or from other skin diseases that have altered the skin surface—for example, burns, poison ivy, eczema, and athlete's foot.

Types of Bacterial Skin Infections

Impetigo

Impetigo is an infection of the skin surface and some of the underlying tissues. It is most common in grade school children and amateur wrestlers.

This infection is characterized by small red spots that occur in clusters on the skin. These fill with yellowish fluid, forming blisters. The blisters eventually burst, leaving yellow or brown crusts.

Impetigo is highly contagious and can spread havoc through a family or classroom. The fluid in the blisters is loaded with bacteria and is often involved in spreading the infection to others.

Most cases of impetigo are self-limited; they go away without treatment within two or three weeks. But some cases progress to the point where they cause serious complications. In a small percentage of infections, the bacteria dig down through the skin and get into the blood, causing septicemia (blood poisoning). They can also damage the lungs, ears, kidneys, bones, and even the heart.

Although most cases of impetigo present no problem, you should never self-treat it. Besides, proper treatment from your doctor can limit the infection to a few days rather than weeks.

Boils and Carbuncles

A boil, more properly called a furuncle, starts as an infection of a hair follicle that invades the lower layers of skin; a carbuncle is an area where several boils have coalesced to form one large infection.

Boils are more common in men than in women and occur primarily in hair areas where there is friction. The neck, waist, buttocks, and thighs are most often involved.

"Drawing" ointments are commonly used to treat boils. These ointments irritate the boil, causing it to form pus at a faster rate than it normally would. The pus accumulation increases the pressure inside the boil and causes it to burst.

Drawing ointments can be dangerous. They not only delay proper treatment from a physician, but they also force the pus and bacteria down deeper into the skin, and possibly into the bloodstream. Once these bacteria get into the blood, they can infect any organ in the body.

Boils and carbuncles should never be self-treated. Your doctor can prevent complications by lancing and cleaning your boils.

Preventing Infection

You should not try to self-medicate any but the most minor skin infection, but you can prevent most of them.

Any cut or abrasion or burn on the skin can be contaminated with bacteria and develop into an infection. With adequate cleansing, however, you can prevent this complication.

Washing with soap and water is one of the safest and most effective first aid infection preventives. Soap doesn't have much antibacterial activity unless it contains an antiseptic like triclosan or triclocarban. Soap's real value lies in the fact that it physically removes dirt, debris, and bacteria from the wound site. Clean wounds seldom become infected.

Several good and not-so-good antiseptics are available for use after the wound has been cleaned properly. Antiseptics differ from disinfectants in that antiseptics are intended for use on the skin; disinfectants are used on nonliving objects like floors, walls, sinks, and toilets.

Antiseptics are designed to be minimally irritating to injured skin, although that's hard to explain to a four-year-old.

Alcohols—Limited by Evaporation

The two most effective antiseptic alcohols are ethyl (grain) alcohol and isopropyl (rubbing) alcohol, but they have their limitations.

Alcohols evaporate quickly and this limits their effectiveness. To have maximum effect, they need to be rubbed onto the skin for at least two minutes. The real problem is holding anybody down that long.

Isopropyl alcohol is probably a little more effective than ethyl alcohol. However, neither type kills viruses, fungi, or bacteria spores. Nor do they have long-lasting effects. Once they evaporate, that's it.

Iodine—An Effective Traditional Antiseptic

Iodine is also a highly effective and time-honored antiseptic. Iodine is available in several forms: iodine tincture, iodine solution, and iodophore. Each has its own particular advantages and disadvantages.

Iodine tincture is a solution of iodine in alcohol. It is the most effective of all the iodine antiseptics, but it also burns like fire. Iodine tincture takes advantage of the antibacterial actions of both iodine and alcohol.

Iodine solution contains no alcohol and is not as effective as iodine tincture. But it doesn't sting as much, either. It's a good alternative for youngsters who run the other way when you pull out the iodine tincture bottle.

Iodophores cause even less irritation than iodine solution, but they are not as effective against bacteria as the other forms. The most commonly used iodophore is povidone iodine, the active ingredient in Betadine. Iodophores are also easier to wash out of your clothes when you spill the liquid on yourself while trying to wrestle a child into submission.

Hydrogen Peroxide—Effective but Brief

Hydrogen peroxide is an old, but effective antiseptic. And it's entertaining, too. Douse your cut with peroxide and listen to it fizz. The noise is caused by the release of a chemically active form of oxygen that butchers most species of bacteria.

Peroxide shares a limitation with alcohol in that it leaves no residue on the skin. Once the oxygen is gone, the drug's activity ends. Most other antiseptics stay on the skin until they either wear off or are washed off.

Chlorhexidine—Excellent Cleansing Qualities

Chlorhexidine is the newest OTC antiseptic. It is available in Hibiclens and Hibistat soaps. It is an excellent cleanser for wounds, but beware. Hibistat contains alcohol and may sting an open wound.

Besides being an effective antibacterial, chlorhexidine has the advantages of poor absorption through intact skin (therefore less chance of side effects), and it forms an antiseptic residue on the skin. The residue continues to kill bacteria until it wears away.

Unfortunately, not all antiseptics are as effective as those just described.

Boric Acid—Of Little Benefit and Dangerous

Boric acid has minor value as an antiseptic but has tremendous potential as a poison. It is extremely dangerous to keep around the house. If it is accidentally swallowed it can cause vomiting, diarrhea, kidney damage, and heart failure. It can also cause severe rashes when applied to the skin.

Boric acid has no significant advantage over any other

antiseptic. Don't let this stuff into your house. Throw it out if it is already there.

Mercurials—Not Effective Against Bacteria

The mercurial antiseptics merbromin and thimerosol, better known by their brand names Mercurochrome and Merthiolate, have been around forever. But longevity isn't a measure of efficacy.

As early as the 1940s there were indications that mercurials only temporarily stunned bacteria; they couldn't kill them. That doesn't sound like a ringing endorsement for an antiseptic.

The mercurials also have the potential to cause more side effects than other antiseptics. While the amounts applied to small cuts and scrapes don't represent a significant hazard, applications over large areas or repeated applications can cause mercury to be absorbed and accumulate in the kidneys and other organs.

More effective and safer antiseptics are available. Why take chances on the mercurials?

Quarternary Ammonium Compounds—Neutralized by Soap

Benzalkonium chloride (Bactine, Mercurochrome II, Zephiran) is the most commonly used compound of this class. Benzalkonium is a fairly good antiseptic, but it has one limitation—soap destroys its antiseptic activity.

If you wash a wound before using benzalkonium, you must remove *all* traces of soap. That means rinsing thoroughly with water followed by alcohol.

If you're going to go through all of that, why not just use alcohol as your antiseptic to begin with and forget about the benzalkonium?

Topical Antibiotics—Relatively Ineffective

Topical antibiotics, the kind you rub onto your skin, can be sold over the counter. But don't get too excited. They aren't all that great.

The FDA advisory panel found that there is little evidence to indicate that these drugs are highly effective. One of the problems is that they can't get as far down into the skin as the bacteria can. There is no proof that you heal faster with antibiotic ointments than you would with time alone.

Antibiotics can also cause allergic skin reactions. If you insist on using an antibiotic, at least pick one that doesn't contain neomycin. As many as one out of twelve people are allergic to neomycin, and indications are that the more often you use it, the more likely you are to have a reaction.

The Pharmacist's Prescription for Skin Infections

Prevention is the best treatment. Wash wounds with soap and water. If the wound was contaminated with dirt or other material, use an effective antiseptic.

Watch any skin disorder for any sign of infection.

Don't try to self-medicate any skin infection.

See the Doctor if . . .
- You show any signs of skin infection, including redness, pus formation, warmth at the site, or swelling.
- You have a wound that seems to heal too slowly.
- You have diabetes or a circulatory problem.

Effective Antiseptics
Alcohol	Iodine tincture
Betadine solution	Isodine Antiseptic
Hibiclens	Solution
Hibistat	Poviderm
Iodine solution	

Or the generic equivalent of any of the above

Antiseptics Not Recommended for Self-Medication
Bactine (B)	Merthiolate (B)
Mercurochrome (B)	S.T. 37 (B)
Mercurochrome II (B)	Zephiran (B)

Or the generic equivalent of any of the above

The products listed in the "Not Recommended" tables are not recommended by me for one or more of the following reasons: (A) One or more ingredients have been reported to be ineffective or only slightly effective for the product's intended purpose; (B) a more effective product is available; (C) the product advertising or description is likely to heighten consumer expectation beyond actual effectiveness; (D) the product has the potential to cause side effects in the average consumer that are more serious than those generally associated with OTC drugs; (E) the product has the potential to cause serious side effects in persons with specific diseases or disorders; (F) another product is available that is capable of producing the same or nearly the same therapeutic effect without the same risk of side effects; (G) persistent use of the product may cause physical dependency that alters an otherwise normal body function; (H) the product's formulation may reduce the effectiveness of one of its ingredients; (I) this is a multiple-ingredient product that may have no therapeutic advantage over simpler or single-ingredient products; (J) one or more of the product's ingredients may be useful for only a short period during the total duration of the illness; (K) the product cannot easily be administered at a dosage level within generally recommended boundaries of optimal therapeutic effect; (L) this is a condition-specific product that is appropriate for use only after a health professional has helped the patient establish a diagnosis.

Athlete's Foot

Athlete's foot is a sexist disease. It occurs almost seven times as often in men as in women.

Athlete's foot is an infection, but it isn't started by bacteria. It begins as a fungal disease. Fungi are microscopic plants that grow as parasites on other living matter.

The disorder is characterized by small blisters and splits in the skin of the foot. The combination of the skin damage and the fungal infestation causes burning, itching, and stinging in the affected areas. If the infection isn't checked, it can spread completely across the bottom of the foot, over to the top of the foot, up the leg, and down into the toenails.

The fungus that causes athlete's foot is the same one that causes ringworm and jock itch on other parts of the body. (Consequently you can use athlete's foot products to treat these disorders.) These fungi love moisture, and the foot is the perfect environment for them. Your feet contain 250,000 sweat glands, all pumping their little hearts out every minute. Each day these little guys dump eight ounces of sweat into your socks. Stuff these glands into a shoe and what could be a better place for fungi to grow and prosper?

Fungal infections are bad enough, but fungi are to athlete's foot what a blasting cap is to exploding dynamite.

The fungi get things started; bacteria pick up the act from there.

Bacteria find their way into the cracks and crevices formed by the fungi and cause the sore to fester. The best treatment, therefore, is aimed at eliminating both the fungi and the bacteria.

How to Treat Athlete's Foot

Lack of proper follow-up is one of the most common reasons for treatment failure in athlete's foot. Most people have no idea how long it takes to get rid of it. Mild cases commonly take two or three weeks of consistent treatment before the fungus is eradicated, and even then it may come back.

You can also reinfect yourself. You can pick it up again in your shower, in the locker room, or even in your own shoes. Shoes can harbor the fungus so that you get a fresh dose of disease every time you put them back on. Actually, the amazing thing about athlete's foot is not that it recurs, but that you ever get rid of it.

The proper treatment of athlete's foot revolves around two factors: foot hygiene and antifungal drug treatment.

The Importance of Foot Hygiene

Mild athlete's foot infections may improve significantly if you just pay close attention to your feet. The single most important thing you can do for your feet is to keep them clean and dry.

Keeping your feet dry includes being careful of what you put on them. Start by changing your socks at least once a day and use absorbent cotton socks rather than synthetics. Kick your shoes off when you're at home in the evening. This helps evaporate the sweat on your feet and makes them less hospitable to fungi.

Your shoes are also important. Avoid shoes that don't let your feet "breathe." These include rubber boots and rubber-soled tennis or jogging shoes. Don't wear the same pair of shoes two days in a row. Alternating days allows the insides to dry out and reduces the number of fungi lurking there.

Wash your feet once or twice a day with soap and water,

but be gentle. You don't have to scrub hard or dig down between the toes. Vigorous washing can damage the skin and allow the fungi and bacteria to get into new areas.

Dust your feet with powder after you wash them. Be sure to get the spaces between the toes with talc or a commercial athlete's foot powder like Tinactin, Desenex, or Micatin.

Medications for Athlete's Foot

While there are dozens of products on the market, most of them use one of three basic ingredients: undecylenic acid, tolnaftate, or miconazole.

These three drugs are true antifungal agents. That distinction separates them from earlier drugs, some of which are still on the market, that simply cause your skin to peel. The theory behind skin peeling agents is that they make the foot less hospitable for the athlete's foot fungus. With the development of effective antifungals, these peeling agents have limited usefulness.

Undecylenic acid. Undecylenic acid and its first cousin zinc undecylenate are the oldest of the three antifungals. Undecylenic acid causes relatively little irritation to the skin or any other side effects, but it isn't terribly effective either.

Undecylenic acid in combination with sweat, fungi, and dead skin on the foot imparts an undescribable odor. Some people get fed up with the stench and discontinue treatment too early. This unfortunately leads to relapse and necessitates retreatment.

Tolnaftate. Tolnaftate is a good alternative for those who can't tolerate undecylenic acid. Side effects from tolnaftate are rare and usually consist only of mild irritation to the skin.

One major limitation of both undecylenic acid and tolnaftate is that neither one has significant antibacterial activity. This reduces their effectiveness on broken or macerated skin.

Miconazole. Miconazole is the cream (or ointment) of the crop. This drug is not only antifungal, but also has some antibacterial activity. It is a superior drug for the treatment of athlete's foot and other fungal infections. Until recently it was available only with a prescription, but it is now available over the counter.

Miconazole and the other antifungals should be applied once or twice daily for several weeks. You should expect to use any of these drugs for at least three weeks before you see much improvement. An advantage of miconazole is that it relieves itching within a few days, while the other drugs may not.

Antifungal agents are sold in a variety of dosage forms: aerosol powders or liquids, creams, gels, liquids, foams, or ointments. Of these, the most useful are the powders, liquids, and creams.

Powders are used primarily as drying agents; they absorb some of the excess moisture around the foot. I normally recommend that people use them after washing their feet. Another way to use them is to sprinkle a small amount inside your socks in the morning. This helps to keep the feet dry longer.

Liquids are probably the most effective form of treatment. Liquids can penetrate deeper into the skin and into the cracks and fissures that may be on the bottom of the feet and between the toes.

Read labels well before you buy a liquid antifungal. Some of them contain alcohol. Slapping alcohol on your sore feet in the morning can wake you up as your morning coffee never did.

Creams are the most popular form of antifungals, and they have a definite advantage. A cream or ointment stays where you put it. It sticks to the infected area and stays in contact with the lesion for several hours. But creams also have the disadvantage of feeling squishy.

Some people declare all-out war on their athlete's foot. They wash their feet twice a day with an antifungal soap, powder up with an antifungal after washing, use a cream at bedtime, and apply a liquid in the morning. This regimen is effective but expensive. Unless you have a raging case of athlete's foot, you probably don't have to go to all that trouble. And if your problem is that bad, you should be seeing a doctor.

The Pharmacist's Prescription for Athlete's Foot

General Information
Keeping your feet clean and dry is the most effective preventive measure.

Laundering socks and bed linens frequently is another recommended preventive measure.

Recommended Treatment
Select an effective antifungal agent and follow label directions.

Use your antifungal regularly for a minimum of two weeks, and probably as long as four weeks or more.

Continue to treat yourself for several days after all signs of athlete's foot are gone.

See the Doctor if . . .
- You have diabetes.
- You have any circulatory problems in your feet or legs.
- Your toenails are involved.
- Your skin has white, soggy patches.
- Your foot oozes fluid or is seriously inflamed.
- Your foot begins to swell.

Products Recommended for Athlete's Foot

Miconazole
  Micatin

Tolnaftate
  Aftate
  Dr. Scholl's
  Foot Work
  Pro Comfort
  Tinactin

Undecylenic acid
  Caldesene Medicated
    Powder
  Desenex
  NP 27 Aerosol
  Quinsana Plus
    Medicated Foot
    Powder
  Ting Powder

  Or the generic equivalent of any of the above

Products Not Recommended for Athlete's Foot

NP 27 Cream (I)   Sopronol (B,I)
NP 27 Powder (I)   Ting Cream (I)
NP 27 Liquid (I)

    Or the generic equivalent of any of the above

The products listed in the "Not Recommended" tables are not recommended by
me for one or more of the following reasons: (A) One or more ingredients have been
reported to be ineffective or only slightly effective for the product's intended purpose; (B) a more effective product is available; (C) the product advertising or description is likely to heighten consumer expectation beyond actual effectiveness; (D)
the product has the potential to cause side effects in the average consumer that are
more serious than those generally associated with OTC drugs; (E) the product has
the potential to cause serious side effects in persons with specific diseases or
disorders; (F) another product is available that is capable of producing the same or
nearly the same therapeutic effect without the same risk of side effects; (G) persistent use of the product may cause physical dependency that alters an otherwise
normal body function; (H) the product's formulation may reduce the effectiveness
of one of its ingredients; (I) this is a multiple-ingredient product that may have no
therapeutic advantage over simpler or single-ingredient products; (J) one or more
of the product's ingredients may be useful for only a short period during the total
duration of the illness; (K) the product cannot easily be administered at a dosage
level within generally recommended boundaries of optimal therapeutic effect; (L)
this is a condition-specific product that is appropriate for use only after a health
professional has helped the patient establish a diagnosis.

Cold Sores

We need to take a little time to discuss cold sores, not
because there are effective OTC treatments for them, but
because the products currently on the market do such a
poor job.

Cold sores, properly called *herpes simplex labialis,* are
among the most common viral infections in this country.
Once you are infected, the virus lives in your nervous
system for the rest of your life. It may reappear as a cold
sore whenever you experience emotional or physical stress.
Cold sores can pop up as a result of sunburns, infections,
menstrual periods, anxiety, depression, fever (hence the
term *fever blister*), or any other stressful state.

The cold sore usually announces its appearance with
intense pain or itching and swelling on or near the lips. It

may also show up inside the mouth. There may be one or more sores present at any one time. They usually start as small blisters that burst and form a yellow crust.

Cold sores are contagious. If you are infected, avoid physical contact with others who may not have been exposed to them previously, particularly children. People who experience their first herpes infection can become extremely ill with high fever and intense pain for up to two weeks.

There is no good way to prevent cold sores from recurring. One possible treatment involves holding ice on the emerging sore for up to two hours. However, this works only if the ice is applied at the very first sign of a fever blister, and you also run the risk of developing frostbite on top of your cold sore.

The Treatment of Cold Sores

No OTC treatment makes a cold sore go away faster than nature itself. Even prescription drugs do a poor job. The best you can hope for is some symptomatic relief. If the treatment you are using doesn't improve your condition or if the treatment makes it worse, stop it immediately and call your pharmacist or doctor.

Since we can't cure cold sores, we have to lower our sights. Our goal in treating them is limited to reducing the pain they cause and to eliminating irritants that may prolong their miserable little lives.

Nondrug treatments include rinsing the mouth with lukewarm water or mouthwash as often as possible, avoiding foods that require prolonged chewing, and avoiding citrus fruits and other acids and salts that can irritate the open sores.

Analgesics—For Some Relief of Pain

Common analgesics like aspirin, acetaminophen (Datril, Tylenol), and ibuprofen (Advil, Nuprin) probably give as much pain relief as anything else. While they certainly aren't miracle drugs for cold sores, they may take some of the edge off the pain, and they are effective in reducing fever that may accompany the sores. You can take them while also using some of the following treatments without concern for drug interactions.

Protectants—To Reduce Drying and Cracking

Once the initial blister dries out, emollient creams or plain petrolatum like Vaseline can be used to cover the surface of the cold sore and trap moisture inside. This is beneficial since much of the pain of a cold sore comes from drying and cracking. Protectants don't have any direct effect on the lesion, but they can reduce cracking, bleeding, and scabbing.

Anesthetics—For Topical Pain Relief

Local anesthetics like benzocaine can relieve much of the pain and burning of a cold sore. Benzocaine can be used either as a solution that is applied directly onto the sores or as an ointment or cream. Normally the ointment and cream bases are preferable because they have a protectant effect.

Counter-Irritants—Not Recommended

After the protectants and anesthetics, OTC treatments for cold sores are sorely lacking.

Counter-irritants like menthol and camphor are included in several cold remedies, but their effectiveness in relieving symptoms is not proven. I don't recommend that you use them.

Hydrocortisone—Do Not Use!

The anti-inflammatory drug hydrocortisone may seem to be just the ticket for a red, inflamed cold sore.

Don't try it.

Hydrocortisone works by crippling the immune system. That's all right during an allergic reaction, but it's the last thing you want when you have an infection. *Don't use hydrocortisone for cold sores*—it may make them worse.

Lactobacillus—No Proof of Effectiveness

Some have promoted *Lactobacillus acidophilus* bacteria found in Bacid, Lactinex, and acidophilus milk as a cold sore treatment. They speculate that these bacteria will restore the natural balance between the herpes virus and the normal bacterial flora of the mouth. Unfortunately, there is no proof that this works.

Lysine—No Proof of Effectiveness

Lysine is a naturally occurring amino acid that has grabbed some attention lately. Doses ranging from 300 to 1200 milligrams have been claimed to speed recovery and discourage recurrence. There is no proof for either of these claims.

The Pharmacist's Prescription for Cold Sores

General Information

There are no cold sore cures. The best you can expect is temporary relief.

Recommended Treatment

Oral doses of aspirin, acetaminophen, or ibuprofen may give you some relief.

Apply a local anesthetic product containing benzocaine, preferably in an ointment base.

Discontinue any product that causes increased pain or irritation.

Follow instructions on product labels carefully.

See the Doctor if . . .

- Your cold sore lasts longer than seven days.
- Your cold sore starts to develop yellow pus.

Products Recommended for Cold Sores

Anbesol Gel   Orajel
Lotion-Jel   Rid-A-Pain Gel
Orabase with Benzocaine   Vaseline
  Or the generic equivalent of any of the above

Products Not Recommended for Self-Medication of Cold Sores

Blistex Ointment (I)
Campho-Phenique (I)
Cold Sore Lotion (I)
  Or the generic equivalent of any of the above

The products listed in the "Not Recommended" tables are not recommended by me for one or more of the following reasons: (A) One or more ingredients have been reported to be ineffective or only slightly effective for the product's intended purpose; (B) a more effective product is available; (C) the product advertising or description is likely to heighten consumer expectation beyond actual effectiveness; (D) the product has the potential to cause side effects in the average consumer that are more serious than those generally associated with OTC drugs; (E) the product has the potential to cause serious side effects in persons with specific diseases or disorders; (F) another product is available that is capable of producing the same or nearly the same therapeutic effect without the same risk of side effects; (G) persistent use of the product may cause physical dependency that alters an otherwise normal body function; (H) the product's formulation may reduce the effectiveness of one of its ingredients; (I) this is a multiple-ingredient product that may have no therapeutic advantage over simpler or single-ingredient products; (J) one or more of the product's ingredients may be useful for only a short period during the total duration of the illness; (K) the product cannot easily be administered at a dosage level within generally recommended boundaries of optimal therapeutic effect; (L) this is a condition-specific product that is appropriate for use only after a health professional has helped the patient establish a diagnosis.

Dry Skin

Dry skin is one of the most common, most misunderstood, and most mistreated skin conditions. Dry skin is not only uncomfortable, but allowing it to continue untreated can lead to deterioration of skin function and skin infections.

Your skin isn't a leather awning over your body. It's a living sponge that needs to hold water to live.

Dry skin, or xeroderma, wears many faces. For some, it may appear simply as itching. For others, it may manifest itself as cracks in the fingertips. In still others, it may present as itching, inflammation, or flaking skin. No matter what it looks like, the causes and treatment are usually the same.

If skin cannot maintain an adequate moisture content, it will shrink and crack. The magic number for the skin is 10 percent. As long as the water content of the skin stays at 10 percent or higher, we will have relatively little trouble with dry skin.

But what can cause it to lose water?

Some factors are obvious—for example, malnutrition and dehydration, exposure to chemicals and strong solvents, and some allergy-related skin diseases.

Some others are surprising—saunas and steam baths, swimming, and daily bathing.

But how can exposure to water cause dry skin?

Dry skin is the lack of moisture inside the skin, but that isn't the whole story. In order to maintain that moisture level we have to have an adequate supply of skin oil, sebum, on the surface of the skin.

Sebum acts as a barrier to water evaporation. It traps water inside the skin and keeps it where it belongs. When we overexpose ourselves to water in a swimming pool or elsewhere, the water washes away some of this sebum. Then there is nothing left to impede water loss.

There are still more causes of dry skin. They include environmental relative humidity below 60 percent, exposure to strong winds, repeated wetting and drying of the skin, and rough clothing.

As we age we lose some of our ability to produce sebum. The elderly are, therefore, at greater risk of dry skin than are children and young adults.

The elderly have to be particularly cautious about their skin care. Dry skin can occur anywhere on the body, but the areas to watch most closely are the forearms, lower legs, hands, elbows, and knees.

The Treatment of Dry Skin

If identifying and correcting environmental causes of dry skin doesn't improve your skin condition, you'll have to start an active treatment program.

You can't pour water back into the skin, but you can try to trap what's there. One way to rehydrate your skin is to apply a lubricant or moisturizer after you take your bath or shower.

Lubricants—Helpful Moisture Retainers

Bath oils like Alpha Keri and Sardo are common lubricants. These are oils, most often containing lanolin or mineral oil, that are specially formulated to mix with your bath water. When you bathe in them a thin layer of oil will cover your skin and trap water there. But be careful when you use them; they can make your bathtub treacherously slick. You could end up with a broken arm or leg as a result of trying to relieve your dry skin.

If your skin is in poor condition your doctor may discourage full-body baths. You can still take advantage of the bath oil's effect by mixing a teaspoonful of oil in two ounces of water. Rub this mixture into the affected areas of your skin.

Moisturizers—Old "Standards" May Be the Best

If you're going to go the rubdown route, you may be better off using a product intended for that purpose. These work best if you soak the affected area in water for about ten minutes, gently pat dry with a towel, and immediately apply your lotion before the water has a chance to escape from your skin.

Glycerin is one of the oldest and cheapest moisturizers. Glycerin and rose water combinations have been around for years. But don't rub pure glycerin on your skin. In high concentrations it becomes a drying agent, and that's the last thing you want.

Glycerin is unique in that it pulls water out of the air and then forces it into your skin. It is dermatology's answer to a heat pump. It works best in humid environments but still does a satisfactory job at other times.

Occlusive agents are probably the most common and efficient moisturizers. They lay down a layer of oil on your skin that prevents water evaporation. The most effective one is petrolatum, plain Vaseline. However, most people won't put up with the uncomfortable feeling they get from greasing up with petrolatum.

As an alternative to using pure petrolatum, drug companies have combined it with other ingredients to make lotions that improve the esthetics of the product. But you must pay a price for convenience. While these lotions are more comfortable to use, they don't work as well.

The selection of a good body lotion is both a matter of individual preference and a matter of trial and error. There are no right or wrong choices. If one product doesn't do a satisfactory job, switch to another. Once you find a product that works for you and isn't too greasy, stay with it.

Skin Softeners—Nongreasy Alternatives

Urea and lactic acid are skin softeners that also help to rehydrate dry skin. Urea is expensive but may be an alternative for those who haven't had a satisfactory response to other lotions. These drugs improve skin tone without being greasy.

Anti-Inflammatory Agents—Only for Temporary Relief

Hydrocortisone may be beneficial to those who have significant itching and inflammation because of dry skin. The ointment form is usually more effective than the creams or lotions.

Hydrocortisone should be considered only a temporary, stopgap measure. Anti-inflammatory drugs like hydrocortisone are only symptomatic treatments; they don't get to the cause of the problem, which is dehydration of the skin. They may be used on rare occasions, but should never be applied on a daily basis.

Fad Items—"Unbelievable" Is Right!

When some advertisers claim that their products produce "unbelievable" improvement of dry skin, they're probably right. The results *are* unbelievable.

There is heavy pressure from consumers for new skin care products, and that pressure often translates into the introduction of less than effective products.

One of the problems in evaluating products for dry skin is that some of them improve the appearance and feel of the skin but don't change the water content. If you're dealing with dry skin, it doesn't do a bit of good to make the skin feel smooth and soft if you can't improve its hydration.

Ingredients that fall into this category include "natural" products like vitamins A, D, and E, as well as elastin, aloe vera, "natural moisturizing factor" (NMF), and mink, avocado, and jojoba oils.

Beware of anything called a "gel." Gels typically have a high alcohol content, and alcohol is one of the worst things you can put on dry skin. Alcohol dissolves the protective oils on the skin's surface and increases water loss.

Soaps and Bathing—A Potential Double Whammy

The combination of soap and bathing is a double whammy for those with severe dry skin. Sitting in a tub or standing in a shower allows water to slowly soak sebum off your skin. Soap chemically strips it off; bubble baths are even worse.

Full-body baths are a special problem for the elderly, who produce less sebum than they did when they were younger. They need to protect the skin oil they have left. Contrary to what they may believe, the elderly should take full-body baths only when they are dirty, and usually no more than once or twice a week. It's better to take sponge baths whenever possible.

Anyone with dry skin should spend as little time in the bath as possible and should use a mild nondetergent soap. Some good brands are Basis, Dove, Lowila, and Tone.

When you get out of the tub or shower, dry yourself *gently* by patting dry with a soft towel. Don't rub hard or vigorously. Then apply a moisturizer to all affected areas as soon as possible.

The Pharmacist's Prescription for Dry Skin

Identify environmental factors (for example, low humidity, irritating clothes, dishwashing detergent) that aggravate dry skin, and eliminate those you can.

Limit the number of baths or showers you take and reduce the amount of time you spend in the bath.

Use a mild, nondetergent soap for bathing and hand washing.

Apply a moisturizing cream when you get out of the bath and whenever you wash your hands.

See the Doctor if . . .
- You have dry skin over large areas of your body.
- Your skin doesn't improve with self-treatment.
- Your dry skin develops into a rash.
- Your skin begins to show signs of infection, such as redness, oozing, warmth, or pus.

Effective Dry Skin Products
Bath oils

Alpha Keri	Sardo
Jeri-Bath	Surfol

Creams and lotions

Acid Mantle	Moisturel
Aquacare	Nutraderm
Carmol	Pretty Feet and Hands
Esoterica	Vaseline Dermatology
Jeri-Lotion	Formula
Keri Lotion	Vaseline Intensive Care
LactiCare	Vaseline Pure Petroleum
Lubriderm	Jelly

Or the generic equivalent of any of the above

The products listed in the "Not Recommended" tables are not recommended by me for one or more of the following reasons: (A) One or more ingredients have been reported to be ineffective or only slightly effective for the product's intended purpose; (B) a more effective product is available; (C) the product advertising or description is likely to heighten consumer expectation beyond actual effectiveness; (D) the product has the potential to cause side effects in the average consumer that are more serious than those generally associated with OTC drugs; (E) the product has the potential to cause serious side effects in persons with specific diseases or disorders; (F) another product is available that is capable of producing the same or nearly the same therapeutic effect without the same risk of side effects; (G) persistent use of the product may cause physical dependency that alters an otherwise normal body function; (H) the product's formulation may reduce the effectiveness of one of its ingredients; (I) this is a multiple-ingredient product that may have no therapeutic advantage over simpler or single-ingredient products; (J) one or more of the product's ingredients may be useful for only a short period during the total duration of the illness; (K) the product cannot easily be administered at a dosage level within generally recommended boundaries of optimal therapeutic effect; (L) this is a condition-specific product that is appropriate for use only after a health professional has helped the patient establish a diagnosis.

Dandruff—A Social Embarrassment

Dandruff is the result of the scalp's natural self-cleaning process. Dandruff isn't dirt and it doesn't mean that a person isn't clean.

Dandruff is more common than you think. While it's rare in children and the elderly, as many as two-thirds of the population have occasional trouble with scalp flaking. Anybody can get dandruff; it doesn't mean you're a social misfit.

The cause of visible dandruff is unknown. We do know, however, that our scalps continually shed the dead cells from the top layer of skin. For some, these pieces of skin are too small to be seen. Others aren't so lucky; their skin sheds in larger patches that speckle the hair and sift down to the shoulders.

Dandruff is not a constant condition. Some people have episodes of dandruff and then improve. For most, dandruff is worse in the dry winter months and then takes a turn for the better in the summer.

The only consistent symptom of dandruff is flaking, but some also experience mild itching. We used to think that dandruff was caused by a yeast called *Pityrosporom ovale*, but we now know that isn't the case. Unfortunately, there are still several antidandruff shampoos on the market that contain antimicrobial drugs intended to kill this yeast. None of these ingredients are necessary.

Is It Dandruff or Dermatitis?

Dandruff is a natural condition that causes nothing more than social embarrassment. Seborrheic dermatitis is another story.

Seborrheic dermatitis is often mistaken for dandruff because it also causes scalp flaking. But seborrheic dermatitis is also a disease of the skin that needs more aggressive treatment, preferably by your doctor.

Seborrheic dermatitis is primarily an inflammation of patches of the scalp, but it may also appear on the face, hairy areas on the trunk of the body, or in skin folds, particularly behind the ears. It causes skin to flake from red, inflamed patches in the affected areas, may cause intense itching, and usually gets worse with stress or poor health. While dandruff usually gets better with age, seborrhea can stay with you for life.

It's a good idea to try to differentiate between dandruff and seborrheic dermatitis, since only mild cases of seborrhea respond well to over-the-counter remedies. The special shampoos that are sold for dandruff can also improve the appearance of seborrhea, but they don't alter the course of the disease. If you think you might have seborrheic dermatitis, you should be seeing a doctor for proper treatment.

Treating Dandruff

Shampooing is both a treatment and a cause of dandruff. Regular, nonmedicated shampoos can reduce the severity of dandruff for as long as four days. For many people, simply washing their hair with their favorite shampoo twice a week is enough to sweep away telltale speckles. But overdoing it can also be the cause of dandruff.

All shampoos are detergents. They clean your hair by removing the natural oils that trap dirt. Daily shampooing dries the hair and scalp and chemically induces a continual state of dry skin. And what happens when the skin is too dry? It flakes.

In reality, many people don't need fancy dandruff shampoos. They just need to give their hair a rest. Unless your scalp spouts oil like an Oklahoma gusher, you don't need to shampoo more than every second or third day. If that still doesn't work for you, there are some good alternative shampoos.

Whatever antidandruff shampoo you use, you should be sure to follow label directions carefully. No antidandruff drug can work if it isn't in contact with the scalp, and the longer it stays there the better it works.

It doesn't do much good to lather up and then immediately rinse the medication out of your hair. The contact time, or the amount of time you leave it in your hair, is critical.

Any time you feel that your shampoo is causing you problems or if it seems that it isn't working as well as it used to, switch to another type. It's probably a good idea to change ingredients every few months to insure a continued antidandruff effect.

You may also notice an *increase* in dandruff when you begin using an antidandruff shampoo. That's nothing to be concerned about. It takes a few washings to clear out the old flakes. You should see a considerable improvement during the second week of use.

Zinc Pyrithione—Safe and Effective for Most People

Head and Shoulders, America's self-proclaimed best-selling shampoo, is about the best you can buy over the counter. Its antidandruff ingredient, zinc pyrithione, is as effective as the selenium sulfide in prescription-strength Selsun shampoo but has less potential for side effects.

Both zinc pyrithione and selenium sulfide are cytostatic agents, that is, they reduce the growth rate of scalp skin cells. This causes these cells to live longer and, therefore, reduces skin flaking.

Zinc pyrithione is remarkably safe and effective. Only 5 percent of users fail to improve their dandruff, and less than a half dozen cases of skin rash from its use have been reported in the last twenty years.

Given its track record, zinc pyrithione has to be my first choice for an antidandruff shampoo.

Selenium Sulfide—Effective but . . .

Selenium sulfide, the active ingredient in Selsun Blue, is as effective as zinc pyrithione but has the potential for more side effects.

It wouldn't be fair to make too big a deal out of selenium's side effects, because they don't happen all that often. On the other hand, the potential for side effects is greater than with zinc pyrithione.

Elemental selenium is extremely toxic and can be absorbed through the skin, especially broken or inflamed skin. Fortunately, selenium *sulfide* is relatively insoluble in water, and this chemical characteristic is its saving grace.

Continuous use of selenium sulfide can leave a slight odor on the hair and can also give it an oily appearance. In rare cases, it can leave an orange cast on both natural and dyed hair.

Coal Tar—Effective but Not Esthetic

Coal tar is the oldest and least esthetic of the dandruff remedies, but it's effective.

Coal tar is exactly what the name implies; it's a tar formed from the chemical breakdown of coal. In its natural state it's a black, gooey mess; when it's incorporated into shampoos, it's just black and gooey.

Coal tar would be much more popular if it didn't occasionally discolor the hair and skin and leave you smelling like an oil field. Other than that, it's a good drug. Some of the newer products use more highly refined tar, but some say that they don't work as well as the older ones. In any event, coal tar removes dandruff scales, reduces itching, and decreases cell turnover in affected areas. In addition to treating dandruff, coal tar is often very effective for seborrheic dermatitis.

Some of the disadvantages of coal tar shampoos can be minimized if you rinse your hair thoroughly after shampooing.

Sulfur—Of Little Use by Itself

Sulfur is an old product that probably has little effect on dandruff if used as the sole active ingredient in a shampoo. Most antidandruff shampoos that contain sulfur combine it with salicylic acid or sodium salicylate. The FDA advisory panel approved the combination of sulfur with salicylic acid for this purpose.

Salicylic Acid—A Peeling Agent

Sulfur and salicylic acid are keratolytic, or peeling, agents. They have no effect on controlling the growth of scalp skin layers; they simply loosen dandruff scales so they can be washed away.

Keratolytics work because they irritate the skin. Be sure to keep them from getting into your eyes, nose, and mouth when you shampoo. They may also damage your hair with prolonged use.

℺

The Pharmacist's Prescription for Dandruff

General Information

Environmental factors such as low humidity or personal habits such as overuse of hair dryers and daily shampooing may lead to dry scalp and dandruff. Try to identify and avoid them as preventive measures.

Recommended Treatment

Start using an antidandruff shampoo, preferably one with zinc pyrithione or selenium sulfide, two or three times a week. Follow label directions carefully.

If your dandruff does not improve within three weeks, switch to a product with a different active ingredient.

Avoid getting antidandruff shampoo in your eyes, mouth, or nose. If this should happen, rinse the affected area carefully with cool water.

See the Doctor if . . .

- You have red or scaly patches on your scalp.
- You have flaky skin patches in places other than your scalp.
- Your dandruff doesn't improve or gets worse after three weeks of self-treatment.
- Your scalp itches much of the time.

Effective Antidandruff Shampoos

Zinc pyrithione
   Anti-Dandruff Brylcreem
   Breck One
   Head and Shoulders
   Zincon
Selenium sulfide
   Selsun Blue
   Sul-blue
Coal Tar
   Ionil-T
   Sebutone
   T-Gel
Sulfur and/or Salicylic Acid
   Cuticura Anti-Dandruff Shampoo
   Ionil
   Sebulex
     Or the generic equivalent of any of the above

5

The Ups and Downs of Digestion

Every investigation which is guided by
principles of Nature fixes its ultimate aim
entirely on gratifying the stomach.
—Athenaeus (circa A.D. 200)

In simplest terms, our gastrointestinal tract may be thought
of as a long, hollow food processor. Food is introduced
to the system through the mouth, where our teeth grind it
to a coarse pulp and mix it with saliva, the first of several
digestive juices.

When swallowed, food passes along the tract of the
esophagus, past the lower esophageal sphincter, and into
the stomach. This sphincter is the muscle that prevents
food from heading back north after entering the stomach.
We'll see later that this sphincter plays an important role
in the prevention of heartburn.

Your stomach, while appearing to be only a wide spot
in the intestine, is a remarkably complex organ. The stomach has a surface area of about 900 square yards and daily
secretes about a half gallon of the juices necessary for
digestion. These include hydrochloric acid, intrinsic factor, pepsin, and gastrin.

As your stomach slowly churns and mixes food with
these acids and enzymes, the process of digestion begins
in earnest. But first your stomach has to be protected from
digesting itself.

Special cells lining your stomach and small intestine
secrete a thick mucus material that prevents the corrosive
gastric contents from coming into contact with live cells.
When the system works properly the mucus presents an
effective barrier, but factors such as emotional stress, cig-

arette smoking, excessive coffee drinking, and alcohol ingestion can cause your gastrointestinal tract to produce so much acid and enzyme that the mucus barrier is overwhelmed. The end result of this "stomach abuse" may be a peptic ulcer.

When it leaves your stomach, the food, not totally unrecognizable, passes into your small intestine. The small intestine is much more important than most people give it credit for. This twenty-foot tube is the workhorse of your digestive system.

The stomach only mixes food with digestive juices; the small intestine is the place where the heavy-duty digestion occurs. In addition, the small intestine is responsible for the absorption of the nutrients in food and for retaining waste materials. These wastes are passed on to the large intestine, the garbage dump of the body.

The large intestine, or colon, is about five feet long and has two primary functions. It continues the process of absorbing nutrients, and it acts as a storage place for solid wastes.

In its storage capacity, the colon collects the undigestible or unabsorbable materials in your digestive tract and holds them until there is an amount large enough to be expelled. It also collects bacteria and dead intestinal cells. When a sufficient volume of waste has accumulated and has been formed into a solid stool, peristalsis, a series of muscle contractions, occurs, causing the stool, or feces, to be moved into the rectum and out the anus. At this point you have completed the process of digestion.

Indigestion and Ulcers

Unfortunately, the process of digestion doesn't always work as smoothly as it was intended to work. In fact, Americans will spend about $250 million this year on antacids for stomach-related disorders. Most of these antacids will be used for the short-term treatment of indigestion from overeating or indiscreet drinking. They are also frequently used for the long-term treatment of peptic ulcer disease.

While much of our stomach distress is self-induced, experts estimate that somewhere between 20 and 40 percent of drug side effects occur in the stomach or other parts of the gastrointestinal tract. The digestive system is much more fragile than most people realize.

The most common self-induced stomach disorder is gastroesophageal reflux, also known as indigestion, heartburn, sour stomach, or acid stomach. The most common symptom of gastroesophageal reflux is an intense burning sensation in the chest. The pain may spread to your throat, your arms, and even down into your lower abdomen.

Reflux is a common complaint among otherwise healthy people. About 7 percent of people experience this problem daily, while one-third of the population may have these symptoms at least once a month.

Reflux is due to the improper function of the lower esophageal sphincter, the muscle that is supposed to prevent regurgitation of stomach contents. A weakened sphincter allows stomach acid to splash up into the unprotected esophagus, thus producing acid burns in this sensitive area. While there is no satisfactory explanation for why this occurs, we do have a pretty good idea of some of the factors that make it more likely.

Common Causes of Gastroesophageal Reflux

Alcohol	Lying down after a meal
Bending at the waist	Obesity
Carbonated beverages	Overeating
Chocolate	Smoking
Coffee	Tight-fitting clothing
Fatty foods in the diet	

Certain foods, beverages, physical conditions, and even clothing styles seem to weaken the sphincter and make reflux more probable. Ingestion of fatty foods, chocolate, coffee, and alcohol are associated with sphincter weakening. Experts also estimate that cigarette smoking saps 50 percent of the sphincter's strength.

In women reflux is more common during pregnancy, when the growing fetus compresses the gastrointestinal tract and places back pressure on the stomach. Obesity and clothing that fits tightly around your abdomen cause the same effects.

Posture also plays a part in reflux. Bending over after a meal places inordinate pressure on this small muscle, as does lying down after a meal.

Another source of stomach discomfort is a condition called gastritis. This is a potentially preulcerous condition characterized by an inflammation of the lining of the stomach.

Gastritis is due to a weakness or break in the mucus barrier that protects your stomach lining. We used to think that this was due solely to chronic alcohol abuse, but we now know that gastritis is a fairly common condition. It may be caused by regular aspirin use, by treatment with various prescription drugs, cigarette smoking, or by emotional stress.

Aside from burning pain, the primary symptom of gastritis is bleeding from the stomach. As long as the cause of the gastritis is removed, the condition usually responds spontaneously, and most people are not sick enough to think about going to the doctor.

One of the most dangerous diseases of the upper gastrointestinal tract is peptic ulcer. In some circles, especially among workaholics, ulcers have become a status symbol. In reality, there is nothing desirable about having an ulcer, especially when you consider the potential cost of hospitalization, surgery, drug therapy, and blood transfusions. Peptic ulcers are debilitating and can kill. They are not to be taken lightly.

Most people think of ulcers as occurring in the stomach, but the great majority actually are in the duodenum, the first portion of your small intestine. Basically, an ulcer is a crater in the lining of the intestinal or stomach wall. Although the exact mechanisms have not yet been worked out, it seems that a weakness of the mucus barrier allows the gastrointestinal acids and enzymes to burrow into the unprotected lining tissue. This self-digestive process continues to eat away at the wall of the affected organ, causing burning and pain.

If the process is not arrested by either spontaneous remission or therapy, the ulcer will continue to grow, eating away at blood vessels and muscle tissue. Bleeding develops in addition to the pain. Depending upon the size and numbers of ulcers, the bleeding may cause an acute anemia and could threaten the life of the victim.

If the ulcer is still not checked, it will continue to eat all the way through the intestine and open a hole to the abdominal cavity. Real trouble starts here because partially digested food, acid, enzymes, and bacteria can now spill directly into a very sensitive area of your body. A raging infection can result and the patient's chances of survival plummet.

About 3 million Americans experience a peptic ulcer each year. Of these 2.4 million are duodenal (intestinal) and 600,000 are gastric (stomach) ulcers. Cigarette smoking is associated with an increase in ulcers. Men are at greater risk of both types of ulcers, but as women begin to lead lives more similar to men's, their chances of developing ulcers are catching up to the men's. In addition, ulcers seem to run in families. You are more likely to develop an ulcer if one of your parents has had ulcers.

As far as the patient is concerned, there isn't much difference between a gastric and a duodenal ulcer. The symptoms are nearly identical, and the drugs used in therapy are similar. The differences are important for your doctor, however, because the drug doses and follow-up tests may vary. See your doctor if you have some of the following symptoms; they may indicate the start of an ulcer.

Some Symptoms of an Ulcer

Back pain
Black or tarlike stools
Bloating
Diarrhea
Loss of appetite
Nausea
Pain in the chest or
   abdomen

Pain that can be described
   as aching, burning,
   cramping, dull, or gnawing
Vomitus containing red
   blood or material that is
   black or looks like coffee
   grounds
Weight loss

Antacids—The Most Common OTC Remedies

Antacids are the nonprescription agents most commonly used for the gastrointestinal conditions we have discussed so far.

Only gastroesophageal reflux and acute gastritis without bleeding should be self-treated. While antacids are frequently used in the treatment of peptic ulcers, they should only be used under your doctor's close supervision. Never attempt to self-medicate an ulcer. Self-medication is a dangerous practice and can earn you a direct ticket to the hospital—or worse.

The information on antacids is presented here for two purposes. First, a few doses of a good antacid can help relieve symptoms of reflux. Second, a well-informed ulcer patient *working with his doctor* can select the antacid product that is most likely to provide the most benefit at the lowest cost.

Mainly because of exaggerated advertising claims, people have many misconceptions about antacids and their ingredients. Antacids *do not* coat the stomach or the ulcer sore, and even if they did, the coating effect probably would not improve their therapeutic effect. In addition, antacids *do not* heal ulcers or stop gastroesophageal reflux.

If antacids can't do those things, what can they do?

Antacids do only one thing—they neutralize acid in your stomach and duodenum. This effect allows them to help relieve the pain of reflux and ulcers and to improve the environment for healing. Other than that, they really don't do too much for you.

If that's so, why are they so commonly used?

With the possible exception of a few prescription drugs (Carafate, Tagamet, Zantac), there still isn't anything significantly better for the treatment of these conditions.

The treatment of peptic ulcer is particularly frustrating. The prescription drugs that are most effective for this condition are expensive, and patients tend not to take them properly, often because they can't afford them. To be used effectively, antacids must be taken in doses so large that they also become too expensive for many people. In addition, most antacids taste so bad that many patients can't force themselves to gulp down the required number of ounces as many as seven times a day for six weeks or more.

Although you may not get this impression from television, antacids are extremely simple compounds. There is very little difference in their composition. Virtually all effective antacids contain one or more of the following ingredients: sodium bicarbonate, calcium carbonate, aluminum hydroxide, or a magnesium alkali.

Some antacids also contain extra ingredients, such as simethicone or alginic acid. These and similar ingredients serve no purpose in the treatment of either peptic ulcer or reflux.

Antacid Ingredients
Sodium bicarbonate. Sodium bicarbonate, or bicarbonate of soda, is one of the oldest and fastest acting of the antacids available today. It is somewhat effective for the treatment of reflux but should *never* be used to treat an ulcer.

The two main problems with sodium bicarbonate are its sodium content and its ability to cause metabolic problems.

Bicarb is loaded with sodium and should never be used by people with heart, blood pressure, or kidney problems, by people who have to take water pills to eliminate excess water, by persons on low-salt diets, or by pregnant women.

Most people who take sodium bicarbonate either buy Arm & Hammer at the grocery store or use the fizzy antacids like Alka-Seltzer. The effervescent Alka-Seltzer tablets that you drop in a glass of water ("Plop, plop, fizz, fizz, oh what a relief it is") represent a particularly poor combination of ingredients. Alka-Seltzer contains aspirin, which is a well-known stomach irritant. Giving aspirin to a person who already has stomach trouble is like pouring gasoline on a fire.

Alka-Seltzer has been discussed in many medical, pharmaceutical, and consumer-oriented books and journals over the years and the conclusion is usually the same: This product has no place in the treatment of gastrointestinal problems.

Sodium bicarbonate and products that contain it should

not be used to treat ulcers because of their potential for causing a condition called metabolic alkalosis. This complication can arise from repeated doses of the drug and has the potential for causing serious imbalances in the body's mineral and electrolyte systems.

Calcium carbonate. Calcium carbonate is another old antacid that may be useful for reflux but poses an undue hazard to patients with ulcers.

One or two chewable tablets may help relieve the burning pain of reflux. In fact, I sometimes chew Tums for this problem myself. However, calcium-containing antacids have been associated with one potentially serious side effect in patients with ulcers. It seems that calcium at times causes the stomach to secrete extra acid. This condition, called rebound hyperacidity, leaves the stomach and duodenum more acidic after the antacid passes than they were before treatment.

An additional potential side effect of large or frequent doses of calcium carbonate is constipation. More recent studies, however, indicate that this may not be as much of a problem as originally thought.

Aluminum and magnesium salts. Aluminum and magnesium salts are generally considered to be the mainstays of antacid therapy and are the primary ingredients in products like Gelusil, Maalox, and Mylanta. While these compounds don't neutralize quite as much acid as sodium bicarbonate or calcium carbonate, they do a good job and cause less troublesome side effects.

Aluminum, usually in the hydroxide form, is the least potent of all commercial antacids and is capable of causing some distressing side effects. For instance, aluminum binds phosphate in the bowel and prevents its absorption. Aluminum also causes constipation in most people who take it consistently.

Then what's so great about this stuff?

The advantages of aluminum are seen when it is combined with magnesium salts. Some magnesium salts, such as milk of magnesia and Epsom salts, are intended to be used only as laxatives and should not be used as antacids.

Magnesium salts are effective antacids, but they have

one major drawback—they cause diarrhea in most people who take them.

Do you get the picture?

When the constipating aluminum hydroxide is combined with the diarrhea-producing magnesium salts, the end result is a somewhat balanced effect on the bowel.

As a general rule, equal amounts of aluminum and magnesium balance each other's effects, but this differs with some people. Therefore, some antacid combinations are designed to be slightly constipating for the average person, while others cause loose stools. It is often necessary for an ulcer patient to experiment with various brands of antacids to find the right balance.

Magaldrate. Magaldrate, the active component of Riopan, is a unique compound. Years ago some enterprising pharmaceutical scientists at Ayerst Laboratories managed to combine both aluminum and magnesium in the same molecule. The result is an antacid that acts in two stages. The magnesium portion neutralizes acid quickly, while the aluminum part has more prolonged effect. The combination also poses little problem to the bowel, although some people may still complain of slight diarrhea.

Alginic acid. Alginic acid is a component of the antacid Gaviscon and its generic mimics. Alginic acid is not an antacid and falls into the gimmick category.

The theory behind the inclusion of alginic acid is a good one, as far as theories go. When a dose of Gaviscon is swallowed with a glass of water, a chemical reaction occurs between the other constituents of the antacid and the alginic acid, producing a sodium alginate foam. Once it reaches the stomach, the foam floats on top of the stomach contents. If reflux occurs, it is the foam that is regurgitated into the esophagus, not the more caustic stomach acid. Therefore, there is no pain from the reflux—at least in theory.

Sounds pretty good, doesn't it?

Unfortunately, the system doesn't work nearly as well as it should. When the FDA advisory panel reviewed the effects of Gaviscon, they found insufficient evidence of the efficacy of alginic acid. Consequently, the manufacturer of Gaviscon now lists alginic acid as an *inactive* ingredient.

Simethicone. Simethicone is another example of a highly advertised gimmick. Simethicone is a defoaming agent. In other words, it causes gas bubbles in the gastrointestinal tract to coalesce so they can be expelled easier.

Simethicone can be a valuable drug for people who have recently had intestinal surgery, where gas accumulation can be very painful. However, simethicone has no value as an antacid and may actually reduce the acid-neutralizing effects of aluminum hydroxide. Its primary contribution is to give products a uniqueness upon which advertising executives can exercise their imagination.

Based on the advertising they have seen, some people believe that simethicone can prevent intestinal gas. In fact, simethicone has the opposite effect. Simethicone causes gas to form larger bubbles that are easier to pass. When it works properly, the result is actually more public embarrassment, not less.

Many experts agree that simethicone does not belong in antacid products.

Antacid Dosage Forms

Antacids are available in a variety of dosage forms, including liquids, powders, chewable tablets, chewing gums, and effervescent tablets. The most commonly used are the liquids and the chewable tablets.

Chewable tablets offer the convenience of portability. It's much easier to carry a few tablets around in your pocket or purse than it is to carry a jug of your favorite liquid chalk. But the advantage of tablets over liquids ends there.

The Acid-Neutralizing Capacity of Some Antacids

Liquid Antacids

Antacid	Relative Potency*	Antacid	Relative Potency*
AlternaGel	6	Kolantyl Gel	10.5
Aludrox	14	Maalox	13.5
Amphojel	6.5	Maalox Plus	13.5
Basaljel	14	Maalox TC	28.3
Basaljel Extra Strength	22	Mylanta	12.7
Bisodol	15	Mylanta II	25.4
Camalox	18	Phosphaljel	2.8
Delcid	42	Riopan	15
Di-Gel	18	Riopan Plus	15
Gelusil	12	Silain-Gelc	59
Gelusil M	15	Titralac	96
Gelusil II	24	WinGel	11.6

Antacid Tablets

Antacid	Relative Potency	Antacid	Relative Potency
Alka-Seltzer Effervescent	10.6	Maalox #1	8.5
Aludrox	11.5	Maalox #2	18
Camalox	18	Mylanta	11.5
Gelusil	11	Mylanta II	23
Gelusil M	12.5	Riopan Plus	13.5
Gelusil II	21	Titralac	7.5
Kolantyl	10.8	Tums	10
Maalox Plus	8.5	WinGel	12.3

*The higher the potency number, the more acid a standard dose of antacid can neutralize.

The antacids that have *the smallest* drug particle size neutralize *the most* acid. Liquid antacids are milled into extremely small particles and then suspended in water. All you need to do is to shake well and swallow. The antacid then goes to work.

Chewable tablets can't be milled the same way or they wouldn't hold together. You have to activate the drug yourself by chewing it into the smallest particles possible. Unfortunately, your teeth can't begin to match the efficiency of a pharmaceutical grinder.

Consequently, antacid tablets aren't as effective as liquid antacids, even if they contain the same amount of active ingredients. The problem is compounded by the fact that some of the newer liquid antacids are being formulated in "double" strengths. For instance, an ulcer patient who is instructed to take a two-ounce dose of Gelusil II liquid would have to chew at least fifteen Gelusil tablets to get the same effect!

Are all liquid antacids the same? Definitely not!

Since all antacids have different ingredients and different concentrations of those ingredients, they also have different levels of effectiveness. For instance, Maalox TC neutralizes ten times as much acid as the same amount of Phosphaljel. Or stated another way, you would have to drink *five ounces* of Phosphaljel to destroy as much acid as you would with a tablespoonful of Maalox TC.

To make matters worse, the FDA doesn't allow manufacturers to list their products' neutralizing capacities on product labels because the Feds feel that this might be "confusing" to consumers.

Balderdash! There is nothing confusing about it. The only caution, however, is that you cannot compare the acid neutralizing potential of tablets with that of liquids. The information listed on page 171 can be used to compare liquids with other liquids or tablets with other tablets. Remember, the antacid in the tablets is not completely utilized.

The comparisons in the table are important for persons with peptic ulcers. While your doctor will select a dose that is appropriate for you, the average person with an ulcer needs to take enough antacid to neutralize about 145 milliequivalents of acid *seven* times a day! When you consider the volume of antacid that you will have to take, plus the cost of the various products, it is important to know about these differences.

For example, the five most potent antacids would cost you $55 to $85 per month if you take the dose described above. The five least potent antacids would cost you between $90 and $750 to get the same effect!

Between the cost and the chalky taste of these drugs it's a wonder that anyone is able to finish a full course of treatment.

Antacid Side Effects

Antacids are not innocuous drugs. I referred to some of their effects on the bowels and metabolism earlier. In addition, they have been shown to interact with a wide variety of other drugs. In most cases antacids *decrease the absorption* of other drugs, resulting in reduced effect of the second drug. Some of these interactions are listed in the table below.

Drug Interactions with Antacids

Antacids may *decrease* the effects of the following drugs:
> Antibiotics, especially tetracycline
> Aspirin
> Digoxin (Lanoxin)
> Indomethacin (Indocin)
> Iron
> Isoniazid
> Levodopa (Dopar, Larodopa, Sinemet)
> Propranolol (Inderal)

Antacids may *increase* the effects of the following drugs:
> Quinidine (Quinaglute and many other brands)
> Warfarin (Coumadin)

Consult your pharmacist or doctor if you must take any of these interacting medications.

Food and Ulcers

In addition to taking antacids for their ulcers, many people place themselves on special diets. Bland diets seem to be a time-honored tradition for treatment of ulcers. Unfortunately, they have no value.

The best advice about diets and ulcers is to avoid foods that you know bother your stomach. Period.

There is no evidence that spicy foods or pepper irritate an ulcer. On the other hand, if you know that anchovy pizzas or barbecued potato chips or certain fast foods burn your gut, don't eat them.

Interestingly, one proven dietary irritant is coffee. And it doesn't seem to matter whether it contains caffeine or not. The ulcer patient should also avoid all alcoholic beverages and stop smoking, preferably permanently.

The Pharmacist's Prescription for Gastroesophageal Reflux

General Information

In some instances reflux can be prevented by:

  Stopping or reducing cigarette smoking
  Eating smaller meals
  Avoiding lying down after a meal
  Elevating the head of the bed at night
  Losing weight, if you are overweight
  Wearing loose-fitting clothes
  Avoiding bedtime or midnight snacks
  Avoiding such foods and beverages that are likely to make reflux worse, such as:
    Chocolate
    Coffee
    Alcohol
    Carbonated drinks
    Foods with high fat content

Recommended Treatment

There is no definitive treatment for reflux, but antacids may be beneficial.

Consult your pharmacist or doctor before self-medicating, particularly if you are on a salt-restricted diet, have heart or kidney disease, or are pregnant.

Choose an antacid that has a good acid-neutralizing capacity and acceptable taste.

See the Doctor if . . .
- You have intense pain in the stomach area or pain that reaches around your back or down your arm.
- You have a crushing pain in your chest.
- You have weight loss resulting from prolonged lack of appetite, nausea, or vomiting.
- You have not received relief from antacids, or you have had to take antacids for more than one week.
- You have vomit that looks black or bloody or looks like coffee grounds.
- You have unusual fatigue, breathlessness, sweating, or chest pain.
- You have any pain in the stomach area that lasts for more than two weeks.
- You have stomach pain that awakens you during the night.
- You have stomach pain that is relieved when you eat.
- You have stomach pain and you have family members that have had ulcers.

Antacids Recommended for Gastroesophageal Reflux

Alka-2 Chewable Tablets	Maalox
Aludrox	Maalox TC
Camalox	Riopan
Chooz	Rolaids
Creamalin	Titralac
Delcid	Tums
Dicarbosil	WinGel

Or the generic equivalent of any of the above

Antacids Not Recommended for Self-Medication of Gastroesophageal Reflux

Alka-Seltzer Effervescent
 Tablets (E,H)
Bisodol Powder (E)
Gaviscon (C)

Gaviscon-2 (C)
Milk of magnesia (F)
Soda Mint (E)
Sodium bicarbonate (E)

Or the generic equivalent of any of the above

The products listed in the "Not Recommended" tables are not recommended by me for one or more of the following reasons: (A) One or more ingredients have been reported to be ineffective or only slightly effective for the product's intended purpose; (B) a more effective product is available; (C) the product advertising or description is likely to heighten consumer expectation beyond actual effectiveness; (D) the product has the potential to cause side effects in the average consumer that are more serious than those generally associated with OTC drugs; (E) the product has the potential to cause serious side effects in persons with specific diseases or disorders; (F) another product is available that is capable of producing the same or nearly the same therapeutic effect without the same risk of side effects; (G) persistent use of the product may cause physical dependency that alters an otherwise normal body function; (H) the product's formulation may reduce the effectiveness of one of its ingredients; (I) this is a multiple-ingredient product that may have no therapeutic advantage over simpler or single-ingredient products; (J) one or more of the product's ingredients may be used for only a short period during the total duration of the illness; (H) the product cannot easily be administered at a dosage level within generally recommended boundaries of optimal therapeutic effect; (L) this is a condition-specific product that is appropriate for use only after a health professional has helped the patient establish a diagnosis.

Constipation

For millions of Americans the "Big C" isn't cancer—it's constipation.

Constipation has different meanings for different people. Medical professionals generally consider constipation to be bowel movements that do not occur frequently enough, are too small for the diet ingested, or require too much straining to pass. Too many patients, on the other hand, think that they are constipated if they don't have a bowel movement daily.

Over 98 percent of Americans have normal bowel movements. However, normal can range from three BM's a day to three per week.

The problem is that people who think they are constipated begin to self-medicate and then develop a real problem. Although there are few medical reasons to use laxatives, many people are convinced that they must take their daily "physic" to maintain bowel function.

Millions of advertising dollars are spent to foster this opinion. The veteran television viewer is inundated with ads promoting the idea that his or her bowels should work like a clock, with precise, well-lubricated movements every twenty-four hours.

Ads may also appeal to special groups. There are commercials for "feminine laxatives" and commercials showing contented seniors going about their daily routines.

I suppose everyone experiences feelings of constipation at one time or another, but very few cases need to be treated. First of all, you are not genuinely constipated unless you have symptoms of constipation. And lack of bowel movements doesn't count.

The typical symptoms of real constipation include a feeling of pressure in the abdomen, lack of appetite, loss of energy, and sometimes a dull headache. These are the results of the accumulation of feces in the large intestine.

Constipation isn't a disease, but it may be a symptom of one. Some of the major causes of constipation are listed here. As you can see, constipation may be more complicated than you think.

Some Causes of Constipation

Anal fissure	Kidney disease
Brain tumor	Laxative abuse
Diabetes	Low blood potassium
Diverticulosis	levels
Drugs (wide variety)	Nerve disorders
Excessive blood calcium	Parkinson's disease
levels	Pregnancy
Intestinal obstruction	Spinal cord injury
Irritable bowel syndrome	Thyroid disease

Fortunately, the constipation that most people experience is not the result of serious illness or drug reactions. It can be caused by emotional upset, changes in routine, travel, inactivity, and changes in diet. Ironically, one of the most common causes of constipation in the elderly is the overuse of laxatives!

Cases of simple constipation—that is, constipation that is not caused by drugs or disease—usually can be treated quite adequately without resorting to laxatives. In fact, laxatives should be considered only when all else fails.

Although there are other factors involved, the treatment (and prevention) of constipation revolves around just three factors:

- Fluids
- Diet
- Exercise

Stool is 85 percent water. People who don't drink enough fluids can't properly hydrate their stool. The result is a small, hard stool that is difficult or even painful to pass.

Two-thirds of people surveyed in one poll were not aware that their diet could affect their bowel movements. For adequate laxative effect, an average-sized man needs to consume only 7 grams, or ¼ ounce, of fiber per day!

Wheat bran appears to be the most effective type of fiber, but fiber from fruit, vegetables, and nuts is also beneficial. Even breakfast cereals such as All-Bran, Bran Buds, Nabisco 100% Bran, and others can provide about a third of your daily requirement in a single serving.

Fiber is essential not only because it provides bulk, but also because it holds water in the stool. Individuals who have diets rich in fiber pass larger stools more easily than those who do not.

Exercise doesn't affect the fluid content of the bowel, but it does stimulate the muscles responsible for propulsion of stool through the colon. Walking and jogging are probably the best types of exercise for this purpose, but consult your doctor before starting an exercise program if you have any type of heart, blood vessel, bone, or joint disease.

In addition to fluid, fiber, and exercise, your daily habits can help you train your plumbing to work properly.

The first rule of bowel training is to answer nature's call when it presents itself. Go to the bathroom when you feel the urge. Unfortunately, some people don't consider it polite to have a bowel movement at another person's house.

Somehow, we have allowed etiquette to interfere with common sense. If you need to have a bowel movement away from home, go right ahead and do it. It's better to experience a little embarrassment than to become a laxative junkie.

Try to establish a regular time of day for your bowel movements. Many people feel the urge after a meal or in the morning or at bedtime. If you notice that your body is developing a regular pattern, go with the flow.

And don't hurry. Remember, you are trying to teach your body a new habit. If you get to the bathroom and you can't produce a stool immediately, be patient. Don't sit and strain, but don't rush away either. All good things take time.

Most importantly, forget about that BM a day myth.

Regardless of what I say, I know that a good many people will run directly to the drugstore's laxative shelf at the first hint of constipation. While I suggest that you try natural means first, a discussion of commercial laxatives is necessary for those who insist on taking a drug to produce a natural function.

The Intelligent Use of Laxatives

Over the years, a variety of names have been used to describe laxatives. Included among them are *physics*, *drastics*, *cathartics*, and *evacuants*.

From the Middle Ages through the early twentieth century, cathartic purging and bleeding were thought to cure a variety of illnesses. George Washington's death was hastened by this practice.

In early twentieth-century America it was common practice for families to purge their bowels, often on Saturday night. Even today, people believe that a laxative-assisted bowel movement is more efficient than a natural one.

Because of dietary deficiencies and lack of exercise, the elderly are at greater risk of constipation than the rest of the population. Nearly 50 percent of all elderly persons use laxatives regularly, and persons over seventy years of age use these drugs twice as often as those between forty and fifty years old. Laxatives are also the most frequently prescribed drugs in nursing homes. More than 50 percent of all nursing home residents receive a laxative and 40 percent take more than one! Laxatives represent 15 percent of all prescriptions in those facilities.

While there are limited instances where laxatives may be necessary, significant misunderstandings are still prevalent about the role of these drugs in manipulating bowel functions.

Common Types of Laxatives

If there were such a thing as the ideal laxative, it would mimic the normal defecation process as much as possible. It should not irritate the intestinal tract, should affect only the end of the colon, where feces are collected and stored, and should do its job within a few hours. When the bowel movement has occurred, the bowel should be able to recover its normal function without further doses of laxative.

Bulk-Forming Laxatives—The Preferred Remedy

No laxative meets our criteria for the ideal cathartic. However, bulk-forming laxatives like Metamucil and Naturacil come much closer than any other group. These drugs are the preferred laxatives for most people because they mimic the actions of fiber in the intestine. They are thus the most naturally acting of all the laxatives.

Most of the bulk-forming laxatives come from plant sources—for example, agar, plantago seed, kelp, and plant gums. Others, like methylcellulose and carboxymethyl cellulose, are synthetic. Still others are combined with other types of laxatives. These combinations aren't necessary and I don't recommend them.

The bulk-forming laxatives appear to be especially attractive for persons with low-fiber diets because of the apparent association between low dietary intake of fiber and cancer of the colon. However, bulk-forming laxatives have not yet been proven to prevent this form of cancer.

The main advantages of these laxatives are that they don't cause intestinal cramping, laxative dependence, or lazy bowel syndrome, nor do they interfere with the absorption of nutrients.

These agents are not free of side effects, however.

The main problem they present is the risk of intestinal obstruction and gas formation if they are not diluted properly. Be sure to read the container label carefully before taking a dose. In most cases you need to mix the measured dose in a full twelve-ounce glass of water or juice before taking it. You may also have to drink another glass of water after taking the dose.

If you don't drink enough water, the drug could make your constipation worse!

Failure to mix the drug properly can cause it to swell up in the intestinal tract and cause an obstruction. Intestinal obstructions may require emergency surgery. All bulk laxatives, including bran, can cause obstructions.

Some of these laxatives also have a peculiar property. If you don't swallow them down immediately after preparing your mixture, they turn into a gel that has to be dug out of your glass. Your dose is ruined and you may as well start mixing another one.

As a general rule, bulk-forming laxatives are the best choice for people who need occasional help moving their bowels. However, you should use no laxative routinely without a doctor's supervision.

Stimulant Laxatives—Popular but Not Recommended

The stimulant (also known as contact or irritant) laxatives are among the most popular laxatives because their action occurs most reliably. Their side effects also occur most reliably.

The stimulants, including Dulcolax and Ex-Lax, irritate the intestinal lining and nerves so that the body tries to expel them and the rest of the intestinal contents as fast as possible. All stimulant laxatives are capable of causing severe intestinal cramping, even those advertised on television as "gentle." The stimulants are also the most abused of all laxatives.

Stimulants are popular because they act relatively quickly and thoroughly. And this is part of the problem. Stimulants not only eliminate feces from the intestine, but also water, protein, minerals, and electrolytes in amounts that are excessive.

Even worse, with consistent use, they cause a condition commonly referred to as "cathartic colon." Unlike the bulk-forming laxatives, these stimulant drugs don't retrain the bowel to function normally. Instead, they make the bowel lazy and, when used frequently, they can make it impossible for the bowel to move without assistance.

Stimulants aren't recommended as the initial treatment of constipation, and they should never be used for more than one week. Even then, they are best used under a doctor's supervision.

The response to a stimulant laxative is unpredictable. One of the strongest of these laxatives is bisacodyl, better known as Dulcolax. I know of one woman who had an uncontrollable bowel movement right in the middle of a restaurant a few hours after taking Dulcolax. I also had a former professor who spent four hours in a bathroom with severe abdominal cramps after taking a single dose of the same drug.

Does this sound like a "gentle" laxative to you?

"Gentle, dependable" Ex-Lax is another example of a stimulant laxative. Ex-Lax must be good stuff; after all, can anything in chocolate be bad for you? You're darned right it can.

Phenolphthalein, the active ingredient in Ex-Lax and several other laxatives, can color the urine and stool pink to red under some conditions. While this isn't dangerous, it can give you a tremendous scare.

More importantly, phenolphthalein is capable of causing intestinal cramping, plus at least two separate and distinct types of allergic reactions. One type of reaction causes red spots and splotches on the skin varying in diameter from a couple of millimeters to several inches. The rash may be accompanied by itching and burning, and may even blister and form ulcers. The blisters are most common around the mouth and genitals.

The other type of reaction is even worse. A large dose in a susceptible person may cause severe diarrhea, intestinal cramping, difficulty breathing, and total failure of the circulatory system.

If that's a safe and gentle laxative, I'd rather be constipated.

The dosage forms available present additional hazards. Children frequently mistake Ex-Lax for chocolate candy or chewing gum. I have had to keep children under observation in the hospital emergency room for several hours because of Ex-Lax overdose.

Stimulant laxatives aren't totally without value. For instance, radiologists find them to be effective in cleaning out the bowel prior to X rays. Other than in preparation for medical procedures, I don't believe these laxatives should be used for self-medication, and I don't recommend them in my practice.

Osmotic Laxatives—Also Not Recommended

The osmotic, or saline, laxatives are about as bad as the stimulants. Milk of magnesia is the most commonly used osmotic laxative.

Milk of magnesia is capable of causing intense cramping and frequently produces a watery, explosive stool. In addition, people with kidney diseases have trouble getting rid of the magnesium and can slowly poison themselves with frequent milk of magnesia use.

People who believe the daily bowel movement myth can quickly get themselves into trouble with either stimulant or osmotic laxatives. These drugs work so effectively that they clear out the entire bowel, thereby leaving nothing for tomorrow's elimination. The only way frequent users can produce a BM the following day is to take another dose of the laxative, and the cycle goes on. Eventually, the bowel becomes fatigued from overwork and can't function without assistance from a laxative. When this happens, you need a good doctor to get yourself straightened out again.

Softeners—Only for Special Cases

Stool softeners occupy a middle ground between the bulk-forming laxatives and the stimulants. They aren't as toxic as the stimulants, but they aren't as effective, either. In fact, softeners are often combined with stimulants in laxative products. Peri-Colace is an example.

Docusate, the most commonly used stool softener, is a detergent that mixes water with stools. This increases the size of the stool and facilitates elimination.

Softeners are most useful in people who have difficulty passing stools or in those people who should not strain at elimination. These include persons with heart conditions, hernias, hemorrhoids, and recent surgery or childbirth.

As with most other laxatives, softeners should not be used for more than a week without a doctor's supervision.

Mineral oil, another example of a stool softener, is also a good example of a drug that has outlived its usefulness.

Mineral oil doesn't offer any significant advantage over other laxatives and has several distinct disadvantages. Small amounts of oil are absorbed into the blood and deposited in the lymph nodes, liver, and spleen, where they can initiate foreign body reactions. After a dose, the throat is coated with oil that can eventually find its way to the lungs, causing irritation and coughing. If you gag on the oil, enough can get into your lungs to cause pneumonia.

Mineral oil also traps oil-soluble vitamins in the intestine and prevents them from being absorbed. These include vitamins A, D, E, and K. Of these, the blockage of vitamin K presents the greatest problem, because consistent use of mineral oil can alter the body's blood clotting mechanism, which depends on vitamin K.

Unlike other laxatives, mineral oil seeps from the anus and can soil underwear. This leakage can also irritate the bottom, causing itching and irritating hemorrhoids. Not a pretty picture, is it?

Laxative Dosage Forms

Laxatives are available in a wide variety of dosage forms, including capsules, tablets, effervescent tablets, liquids, suppositories, enemas, chocolate-coated tablets, and chewing gum. The candy-type laxatives present a problem not only with children's overdoses, but also with the fact that many people don't consider them to be drug products. It's tempting to overuse them because drugs in candy form surely can't be harmful.

Enemas are routinely used to clean out hospitalized patients prior to surgery, childbirth, or various rectal or bowel examinations. As a general rule, they should not be used for self-medication. Tap water enemas can produce serious fluid and electrolyte problems. An improperly inserted nozzle can act as a skewer, seriously injuring the unsuspecting target. Soap suds enemas can cause allergic reactions and rectal irritation that can last as long as three weeks.

A commercial enema, Fleet's Phosphate Enema, is loaded with sodium and can exceed a heart or kidney patient's daily salt allotment with a single dose.

The elderly, frequent targets of laxative advertisements, are at the same time the group that should be most cautious about using any laxative at all. Seniors have diminished body fluid reserves and are more sensitive to the metabolic side effects of laxatives and enemas. They are also more likely to gag on mineral oil, to experience magnesium poisoning from milk of magnesia, or to overdose on sodium from packaged sodium phosphate enemas.

Seniors are more likely to have mistaken notions of what proper bowel habits are. They may be more easily talked into using unnecessary laxatives simply because "everyone knows'' that the elderly have trouble moving their bowels.

Children, at the other end of the age spectrum, also are susceptible to laxative toxicities. I can't count all the tap water enemas my well-intentioned grandmother gave me when I was a child. Nor can I forget the doses of Fletcher's Castoria that were poured down my gullet.

It's frustrating to know that these practices still continue in many homes, despite the fact that few children need laxatives. I know a woman who gave her children an enema whenever they had a cold.

The Pharmacist's Prescription for Constipation

As a preventive measure, avoid processed white flour in your diet. Substitute whole wheat. In general it is helpful to avoid low-fiber foods in your diet, including cakes, puddings, candy, and pastry.

Eating extra fruit and vegetables will help promote regular bowel movements.

Establish regular times for bowel movements.

Heed the urge to defecate whenever it presents itself.

Keep track of bowel habits for at least two weeks before deciding you are constipated.

If you feel you are constipated, start with simple corrective efforts first, unless your doctor has advised you otherwise:

Increase your fluid consumption.

Increase the fiber in your diet.

Increase your daily exercise.

If a laxative is necessary, use any of the bulk-forming laxatives included in the list that follows. Follow the dosing and mixing directions on the product label.

See the Doctor if . . .
- Your symptoms have lasted for more than two weeks.
- You had a disease of the gastrointestinal tract prior to the constipation.

- Your constipation comes on suddenly with no apparent cause.
- You experience pain when trying to pass a stool.
- You have blood in your stool, or your stool is dark and tarlike.
- You have abdominal pain, bloating, sudden weight loss, fever, or nausea.
- You feel that you need to use a laxative regularly.

Recommended Laxatives
All are bulk-forming laxatives.

Effersyllium	Mitrolan
L.A. Formula	Modane Bulk
Maltsupex	Mucilose
Metamucil	Naturacil

Or the generic equivalent of any of the above

Laxatives Not Recommended for Self-Medication

Agoral (F,I)	Fleet Pediatric Enema (E)
Agoral Plain (F,I)	Fletcher's Castoria (G)
Alophen (G)	Haley's M-O (G,I)
Bisacodyl (G)	Innerclean Herbal Laxative
Black Draught (G)	(G,I)
Caroid Laxative Tablets	Kondremul (I)
(G,I)	Modane (G)
Carter's Little Pills (G)	Modane Mild (G)
Castor oil (D,G)	Nature's Remedy (G,I)
Colace (B)	Neoloid (D,G)
Correctol (G,I)	Peri-Colace (G,I)
Dialose Plus (G,I)	Petrogalar (F)
Doxidan (G,I)	Phospho-Soda (E)
Doxinate (B)	Senokot (G)
Dr. Caldwell's Senna	Senokot-S (G,I)
Laxative (G)	Stimulax (G,I)
Dulcolax (G)	Surfak (B)
Ex-Lax (G)	Theralax (G)
Feen-A-Mint (G)	
Fleet Enema (E)	

Or the generic equivalent of any of the above

The products listed in the "Not Recommended" tables are not recommended by me for one or more of the following reasons: (A) One or more ingredients have been reported to be ineffective or only slightly effective for the product's intended purpose; (B) a more effective product is available; (C) the product advertising or description is likely to heighten consumer expectation beyond actual effectiveness; (D) the product has the potential to cause side effects in the average consumer that are more serious than those generally associated with OTC drugs; (E) the product has the potential to cause serious side effects in persons with specific diseases or disorders; (F) another product is available that is capable of producing the same or nearly the same therapeutic effect without the same risk of side effects; (G) persistent use of the product may cause physical dependency that alters an otherwise normal body function; (H) the product's formulation may reduce the effectiveness of one of its ingredients; (I) this is a multiple-ingredient product that may have no therapeutic advantage over simpler or single-ingredient products; (J) one or more of the product's ingredients may be used for only a short period during the total duration of the illness; (K) the product cannot easily be administered at a dosage level within generally recommended boundaries of optimal therapeutic effect; (L) this is a condition-specific product that is appropriate for use only after a health professional has helped the patient establish a diagnosis.

Diarrhea

Why do so many people swear by diarrhea remedies that have little or no effect? Because most cases of acute diarrhea, the type that comes on abruptly and remits just as quickly, improve quickly without any treatment at all.

One reason that many people improve so quickly is because they don't really understand what does and doesn't constitute diarrhea.

Diarrhea is characterized by both excessive water in the stool and frequency of stool. Some healthy people may have as many as three stools per day without having diarrhea, while others may have as little as one watery stool per day and have true diarrhea.

The main factor that contributes to diarrhea is a defect in handling the water that is normally reabsorbed into the gut. We usually eliminate two to four ounces of water through bowel movements each day. In typical cases of diarrhea, however, we usually lose seven ounces or more.

Is diarrhea only a nuisance, or can it be dangerous?

We are all acquainted with annoying cases of diarrhea

that accompany the flu. However, most people aren't aware that there are at least fifty medical conditions that may cause diarrhea. Diarrhea may be a symptom of liver, kidney, lung, heart, or thyroid disease. It can also be an early sign of drug toxicity or cancer. In other words, diarrhea may be a tip-off that something serious is happening.

Acute diarrhea may also be caused by nerve disorders, psychological problems, the after-effects of surgery, allergies, intestinal irritants, dietary imbalances, and, of course, infections.

But can diarrhea by itself be dangerous?

You bet it can!

Acute diarrhea can kill a two-month-old infant in as little as twenty-four hours. Diarrhea is *always* dangerous in infants and small children. *Never hesitate to call your doctor if your child has uncontrollable diarrhea.*

Besides being dangerous in children, diarrhea is also common. Acute diarrhea ranks right behind respiratory infections as a common cause of illness in industrial countries.

You've probably noticed that up to this point I've been discussing acute diarrhea. It stands to reason that if there is acute diarrhea, there must also be a chronic form.

Chronic Diarrhea

Chronic diarrhea is more complex than acute diarrhea. This condition is characterized by recurring episodes of diarrhea that usually last for more than two weeks. Like the acute form, chronic diarrhea may be caused by a problem in the bowel itself or may only be a symptom of some other problem.

Even if you feel that you can put up with this problem, you need to get it checked out by a doctor. Over-the-counter medications seldom control chronic diarrhea, and even if they do, a delay in proper diagnosis may cause a worsening of the basic problem. At the very least, chronic diarrhea may cause weight loss or malabsorption of nutrients.

Ironically, one cause of chronic diarrhea is laxative abuse. As hard as it may be to believe, some people over-use laxatives, develop chronic diarrhea, and go to the doctor for treatment. When the doctor questions them about use of medications, including laxatives, these patients may actually deny using these drugs! Why do they bother going to the doctor if they are going to lie about the cause of their problem?

If you feel that you may have chronic diarrhea, go to your doctor. Don't try to self-medicate this condition. For the rest of this section we will discuss forms of acute diarrhea only.

Traveler's Diarrhea

Traveler's diarrhea, also known as *turista* and by many other names (some of them not suitable for a family publication), is a common disorder that usually begins within a few days after arriving in a new locale or a foreign country. It is characterized by violent diarrhea, usually with vomiting and intense intestinal cramps. While there are many treatments or preventives available for this problem, not all cases are preventable.

Some of the common admonitions include avoiding the local water, peeling fruit before eating, avoiding raw vegetables, and making sure all other foods are properly stored, cleaned, and cooked. Food in public cafeterias or from street vendors isn't as safe as that in private homes.

And stay out of swimming pools. I know one family that suffered a ruined Mexican vacation because the hotel pool wasn't properly chlorinated.

The U.S. Food and Drug Administration advises people traveling through areas with poor sanitation to drink only boiled or bottled water, bottled carbonated beverages, or beer or wine.

This isn't always easy to do. Some people take all of these precautions but then brush their teeth with tap water. Or they take ice cubes in their water or cocktails. Despite what some people think, the alcohol in a cocktail doesn't kill the bacteria in the drink.

Even if you do take all the precautions you can think

of, there is no guarantee that you won't get diarrhea.

Your doctor is your best source for prevention of traveler's diarrhea. Certain antibiotics that are available only by prescription seem to be effective preventives. However, two drugs, iodochlorhydroxyquin and diiodohydroxyquin, formerly used for this purpose, have been withdrawn from the market in the United States because of their ability to cause a severe eye disorder.

Some reports in medical journals have indicated that Pepto-Bismol may be an effective over-the-counter preventive for traveler's diarrhea. There are two problems with this treatment. First, it appears that you have to take about eight ounces of Pepto-Bismol each day for this purpose. Second, unlike other products for diarrhea, Pepto-Bismol contains an aspirinlike drug that is the equivalent of about eight aspirin tablets when you take the dose required to prevent traveler's diarrhea. This is a level that can cause serious side effects for some people, especially if they are already taking aspirin for some other condition.

Since your doctor has safer and more effective treatments available, I recommend that you go that route.

It's much better to prevent traveler's diarrhea than to treat it after it occurs. After the onset of illness, the infection has to run its course. Drugs that we normally would use for other types of diarrhea may trap the noxious bacteria in the intestine and make the illness last longer. In many cases, antibiotics either are not helpful, or actually are harmful.

Stricken wayfarers are often tempted to go to the local pharmacy for some symptomatic relief.

Don't do it!

Most foreign countries don't have the strict drug regulations we have in this country. Many potent, potentially dangerous, or potentially ineffective drugs can be sold without prescriptions. If the diarrhea is painful or debilitating, try to get to a doctor and explain your concerns about proper treatment.

Drug-Induced Diarrhea

Before starting your own treatment for diarrhea, remember that many drugs can cause loose bowel movements.

Almost all drugs have been implicated in causing diarrhea and/or constipation. The most common offenders include laxatives and antibiotics, but many others have also been shown to be at fault.

Many laxatives work by forcing more fluid into the bowels to produce a stool. If subsequent doses are taken too soon, however, there may not be enough fibrous waste material in the intestine to soak up the water, and a diarrheal bowel movement may result.

The ability of laxatives to produce diarrhea is related to both the potency of the laxative and the frequency of use. Extremely irritating laxatives may cause diarrhea in as little as two consecutive days of use, while milder laxatives may not produce problems for several days or even weeks.

Antibiotics can cause diarrhea in two days. Since antibiotics kill off bacteria, or flora, indiscriminately, they may alter the intestinal environment. This bacterial massacre may destroy the balance that normally helps to regulate bowel function. Diarrhea frequently results.

In other cases, antibiotics may be irritating to the intestinal wall. The gut responds by trying to expel the irritant along with all the bowel contents. In either case, call your pharmacist or doctor to determine whether you should continue the medication or not.

Antacids that contain too much magnesium, even the drugs you may take for your blood pressure, heart disease, or diabetes, may cause diarrhea.

Likewise, your diet could be the cause of your problem. Foods that contain too much fat, spice, or roughage—or overdoing it with your morning bran—can initiate the trots. Milk or foods made with milk or milk by-products can cause intense diarrhea in susceptible people.

And while we're mentioning food, if one or more friends or family members get diarrhea within a few hours of eating the same food, suspect food poisoning and call your doctor.

The Treatment of Diarrhea

As a general rule, it is better to undertreat than to overtreat diarrhea.

Take your temperature each day that the diarrhea is present and report any fever to your doctor. And drink plenty of fluids. Remember that you lose a lot of water with diarrhea, and you can really get sick if you don't replace this loss. Unless your doctor has restricted your fluid intake, drink at least four glasses of clear liquids every twelve hours.

Some of the things you should *not* do include taking any medication that has not been prescribed for you or has not been recommended by a health care professional. Also, watch your diet. Don't drink milk or eat dairy products. Fresh fruits and vegetables may worsen the diarrhea. Cigarette smoking, coffee, and spicy foods can also increase the frequency of your trips to the toilet.

Remember that diarrhea is only a symptom of illness. Control of the symptom doesn't necessarily mean that the underlying problem has improved.

Despite the fact that there are over a hundred products intended for the relief of diarrhea on the over-the-counter market, only a few of them have shown any benefit after thorough testing. In cases where the diarrhea is caused by something other than a "twenty-four-hour bug," it may be better treated by addressing the underlying cause.

Kaolin-Pectin—Not Proven Effective

If you've ever wondered why Kaopectate and similar products taste like mud, it's because they contain mud.

Kaolin, also known as China clay, is used in many OTC antidiarrheal products to form bulk and to try to trap some of the toxins that cause the diarrhea. Pectin, another common ingredient in these products, is derived from apples and is supposed to form a gel in the intestine.

At best, these products change the appearance of your stool. Other than that, little is known about their effectiveness. The FDA advisory panel reports that, although drugs like Kaopectate and Parepectolin appear to be safe, there is little evidence that they are effective.

Since their efficacy is unproven, these drugs rate a spot on my "Not Recommended for Self-Medication" list.

Bismuth—Not Recommended

Bismuth has been shown to be effective for the prevention and treatment of traveler's diarrhea, but that's it.

Bismuth is an old drug that has outgrown its usefulness. Bismuth is still available in two forms: bismuth subsalicylate and bismuth subnitrate. We've already discussed the problem with the aspirin-like subsalicylate in the section on traveler's diarrhea. (Pepto-Bismol is the brand name usually involved.) The subnitrate may be even more of a problem.

In the intestine, the subnitrate portion of the molecule is converted to nitrate ion. Nitrate is capable of dropping your blood pressure and attacking the hemoglobin in your red blood cells.

Since bismuth compounds are not effective for diarrhea other than traveler's diarrhea, I don't recommend them.

Anticholinergics—Not Recommended and Potentially Toxic

These derivatives of the natural product belladonna have the distinction of being potentially *both* ineffective *and* toxic.

These drugs are capable of reducing diarrhea, but not in the doses available in over-the-counter drugs. The problem is that the effective dose is very close to the toxic dose, especially for children.

Anticholinergics reduce the ability of the colon to move fecal material along its course. This causes the diarrheal stool to stop dead in its tracks, hopefully until the patient regains proper bowel function. However, the doses that are required to do this may also cause blurred vision, dryness of the mouth, painful retention of urine, and flushing of the skin.

Some products like Donnagel combine anticholinergics (belladonna, scopolamine, atropine, hyoscyamine) with kaolin and pectin to try to deliver a therapeutic response by using a combination of several drugs. If the number of ingredients were proof of efficacy, Donnagel would be the drug of choice for diarrhea, instead of just another of my "Not Recommended for Self-Medication" products.

Narcotics—Not Available in Effective Dosages

Narcotics, including paregoric, also work by decreasing the colon's ability to pass stool along its course. The problem with paregoric and the other narcotics is that drug abusers have forced federal regulators to change the laws that govern the sale and use of these drugs. You can no longer buy paregoric without a prescription, except in products that contain ineffective constituents.

Paregoric is effective in doses of one teaspoonful for adults and one-fourth to one-half teaspoonful for children between the ages of six and twelve. Don't take any paregoric-containing drug for more than two days. Paregoric is available over the counter in products like Donnagel-PG.

Paregoric works because of its morphine content. For over a century, morphine has been known to cause constipation and to reduce diarrhea.

There's one more problem with paregoric. While it may relieve the diarrhea and even the abdominal cramping, it appears that it does not decrease fluid loss. This can be an insidious problem. When your diarrhea stops, you may be fooled into thinking that you don't need to keep up your fluid intake.

Bulk-Forming Laxatives—Paradoxically Effective for Diarrhea

Ironically, one of the most effective antidiarrheal agents is a laxative.

Bulk-forming laxatives do the same thing for diarrhea that they do for constipation. In constipation they soak up intestinal fluids to form a larger stool. In diarrhea, they take up some of the excess fluid in the intestine to form a solid or semisolid stool.

While all bulk-formers do this to some extent, polycarbophil is almost four times as efficient as the next best agent. In addition, polycarbophil, the active ingredient in Mitrolan, is one of the few such drugs judged both safe and effective by the FDA advisory panel.

There are a few precautions that you should observe prior to dosing up with Mitrolan. Mitrolan, or any other OTC antidiarrheal, should not be used in children under three years of age. While the drug is not absorbed from the gastrointestinal tract and has few side effects, it can cause serious problems in people with obstructions in their intestinal tracts. Mitrolan can also cause bloating and stomach pain.

Mitrolan doesn't shorten the course of diarrhea, nor does it diminish the fluid loss associated with the illness. It only allows you to pass a semisolid stool. You still need to drink lots of fluids and call your doctor if you don't get better.

Mitrolan tablets should be chewed, not swallowed whole. Be sure to read the directions and dosing information on the package to ensure that you are using it right.

Lactobacillus—A Questionable "Natural" Remedy

The use of *Lactobacillus* bacteria is one of the most controversial forms of diarrhea treatment.

The basic idea sounds pretty good. Ingesting these microorganisms by drinking acidophilus milk or by taking commercial products like Lactinex or Bacid may help to restore the natural flora to an upset intestine. These bacteria are completely safe, but there is no solid evidence that they are effective for diarrhea.

Its proponents argue that *Lactobacillus* is a "natural" remedy and is, therefore, preferable to the synthetic drugs that pharmacists and doctors try to pawn off on you.

While these bacteria may be safe and natural, they don't work. In fact, the logic doesn't even follow. Diarrhea itself is natural, in that it occurs in nature, but we certainly don't want to have it.

The Pharmacist's Prescription for Diarrhea

Watch your fluids. Drink at least four glasses of water every twelve hours, unless your doctor has instructed you otherwise. Do not eat or drink dairy products until you are better.

Avoid any foods that you know are upsetting to your stomach or intestines.

Take your temperature at least once a day.

Ask your pharmacist or doctor if any medications you are taking could be the cause of your diarrhea.

Do not try to treat children under three years of age. Call your doctor for instructions.

See the Doctor if . . .

- You are over sixty years of age and are in poor health.
- You are pregnant.
- You have a chronic disease.
- Your belly feels sore.
- You have a fever.
- You have lost more than 5 percent of your total body weight since the start of the diarrhea.
- Your diarrhea has lasted more than two days, despite treatment.
- You have blood in your stool or your stool looks black.

Products Recommended for Diarrhea

Mitrolan
    Or the generic equivalent

Products Not Recommended for Self-Treatment of Diarrhea

Bacid (A)
Donnagel (A,I)
Donnagel-PG (A,I)
Kaodene Non-Narcotic
    (A)
Kaodene with Paregoric
    (A)

Kaopectate (A)
Kaopectate Concentrate
    (A)
Lactinex (A)
Parepectolin (A)
Pepto-Bismol (E)

Or the generic equivalent of any of the above

The products listed in the ''Not Recommended'' tables are not recommended by me for one or more of the following reasons: (A) One or more ingredients have been reported to be ineffective or only slightly effective for the product's intended purpose; (B) a more effective product is available; (C) the product advertising or description is likely to heighten consumer expectation beyond actual effectiveness; (D) the product has the potential to cause side effects in the average consumer that are more serious than those generally associated with OTC drugs; (E) the product has the potential to cause serious side effects in persons with specific diseases or disorders; (F) another product is available that is capable of producing the same or nearly the same therapeutic effect without the same risk of side effects; (G) persistent use of the product may cause physical dependency that alters an otherwise normal body function; (H) the product's formulation may reduce the effectiveness of one of its ingredients; (I) this is a multiple-ingredient product that may have no therapeutic advantage over simpler or single-ingredient products; (J) one or more of the product's ingredients may be used for only a short period during the total duration of the illness; (K) the product cannot easily be administered at a dosage level within generally recommended boundaries of optimal therapeutic effect; (L) this is a condition-specific product that is appropriate for use only after a health professional has helped the patient establish a diagnosis.

Nausea and Vomiting

What's good for vomiting? Not much.

Vomiting and its predecessor, nausea, are complex processes that involve both the gastrointestinal tract and the central nervous system.

Most people tend to think that only those substances that irritate the stomach can cause vomiting. Actually, most cases of vomiting are initiated either by disturbances in the inner ear or by toxic chemicals in the blood that stimulate a portion of the brain called the chemoreceptor trigger zone.

As obnoxious as it is, vomiting does have a purpose. Vomiting is one means the body has of ridding itself of irritating or dangerous substances. Vomiting protects us from some types of poisons.

Unfortunately, the system sometimes runs amok. In pregnancy, the brain mistakes high hormone levels as a poison and initiates vomiting. The brain, through sensors in the inner ear, also identifies certain types of motion as being dangerous and initiates the urge to upchuck. The medical causes of vomiting are many and varied. Some of the more important ones are listed in the box.

Some Causes of Vomiting

Blood electrolyte imbalances	Infections
Brain tumors	Kidney diseases
Cancer	Liver disease
Diabetes	Migraine headache
Drugs (many types)	Motion
Ear diseases	Overeating
Epileptic seizures	Pain
Fever	Poisoning
Gastrointestinal disorders	Pregnancy
Glaucoma	Psychological stress
Head injuries	Radiation therapy
Heart attack	Thyroid disease
Heart failure	Visual problems
Hypertension	

Aside from the obvious esthetic problems associated with vomiting, there are also medical complications. Most of these are only seen with prolonged vomiting and include blood electrolyte imbalances, dehydration, and kidney problems. Strenuous vomiting can also tear portions of the gastrointestinal tract and may burst blood vessels. Prolonged or repetitive vomiting can even erode the enamel on your teeth.

Most people who are that sick have sense enough to go to the doctor. However, one problem that happens all too often in the elderly and debilitated is aspiration of vomitus. In this case the patient inadvertently gags and sucks vomitus down into the lungs. This causes a dangerous form of pneumonia that is very difficult to treat.

Motion Sickness Remedies

Unfortunately, the only form of nausea and vomiting that we can even halfway treat with over-the-counter drugs is motion sickness. You can experience motion sickness—also known as sea sickness, car sickness, or air sickness—in any situation where movement confuses your body.

Research interest in motion sickness has been sporadic. There was a great effort to find the cause and treatment of this problem during World War II, when the Navy had to transport troops across the oceans. However, when the war ended, the research did, too. Interest picked up again a few years ago when our astronauts started vomiting in small, weightless space capsules.

Various theories have been proposed to explain motion sickness, but there has been little progress in the area of OTC treatments. We are still limited to drugs that were developed thirty years ago.

Everyone is susceptible to motion sickness. Some people just have a greater tolerance for motion than others. There are a few nondrug remedies that you can use to try to prevent this problem. If you have problems with motion sickness, try not to eat large meals before traveling, and try to drink a lot of clear fluids. Water, tea, or noncarbonated soft drinks may be helpful.

Once nausea occurs it is much more difficult to treat. However, lying flat on your back with your eyes open seems to help some people. If you are traveling in an airplane, you may get some relief by focusing your eyes on the horizon. These maneuvers help to decrease the perception of motion.

Motion sickness can also be prevented by medicating yourself about an hour before departure. While several types of OTC drugs have been actively promoted for relief of nausea and vomiting, the only ones that have been proven to work are antihistamines, and even then, they only work for motion sickness.

Antihistamines—Some May Help

Not all antihistamines are effective for motion sickness. The three most effective ones are cyclizine (brand name Marezine), meclizine (brand name Bonine), and dimenhydrinate (brand names Dramamine and Trav-Arex).

Although dimenhydrinate is the most commonly used and most actively advertised of the three, meclizine has one important advantage—it has the longest duration of action and only needs to be taken once a day. The other two have to be taken from two to four times a day to achieve the same effect.

Remember that these drugs should be used only for treatment of motion sickness. They should not be used for morning sickness in pregnancy or for any other type of nausea. They are also capable of causing most of the antihistamine side effects described in chapter 2.

Other OTC Antinauseants

While there are several prescription drugs that are effective for other types of nausea, there really isn't much available on the OTC market.

Pepto-Bismol—Does It Relieve Nausea?

One of the pretenders to the throne is our old friend Pepto-Bismol. Television ads strongly imply that this drug is effective for the nausea that may accompany overeating. Unfortunately, Pepto-Bismol does not reliably relieve the nausea from this or any other condition. In fact, many people have told me that the taste and texture of Pepto-Bismol make them gag.

Pepto-Bismol also has one unique side effect that wasn't mentioned earlier. If used over a long period of time, it can darken your tongue, dentures, and stools!

Phosphorylated Carbohydrate—Not a Proven Remedy for Nausea

Another questionable OTC antinauseant is the so-called phosphorylated carbohydrate. The most common brand name for this compound is Emetrol.

Emetrol is a mixture of the sugars fructose and glucose, with phosphates added. The theory is that this mixture will slow the rate of stomach emptying and thereby reduce the feeling of nausea.

In reality, the stuff has not been proven to work. Also, large doses of fructose can cause abdominal pain and diarrhea. People with poorly controlled diabetes should avoid this drug, since it is capable of significantly increasing a diabetic's blood sugar.

Cola syrup falls into the same category as the phosphorylated carbohydrates, but I have successfully used cola syrup on my own kids. I don't believe that it has any direct effect on nausea in children, but I do find that one or two teaspoonfuls over crushed ice has a pleasant taste that calms the kids down, and that makes them feel a little better.

Cola syrup is available in most pharmacies and is less expensive than any of the other products I have described. If you have children, a four-ounce bottle is a good investment.

The Pharmacist's Prescription for Vomiting

If you are susceptible to motion sickness:
  Avoid large meals before traveling.
  Drink plenty of clear fluids.
  Keep your eyes fixed on the horizon.
  Adults may take 25 to 50 milligrams of meclizine one hour before departing.

See the Doctor if . . .
• Your child is vomiting and is less than one year old.
• Your child is not able to keep fluids down for twelve hours.
• You are physically debilitated.
• You have a fever.
• You have blood or material that looks like coffee grounds in your vomitus.
• Your vomiting lasts more than three days.

- You are pregnant.
- Your vomiting is severe.
- You develop pain in the stomach or belly.
- Your stomach begins to swell.

Recommended for Prevention of Motion Sickness
    Bonine
    Dramamine
    Marezine
    Trav-Arex
      Or the generic equivalent of any of the above

Products Not Recommended for Self-Treatment of Nausea or Vomiting
    Emetrol (A)
    Especol (A)
    Pepto-Bismol (A)
      Or the generic equivalent of any of the above

The products listed in the "Not Recommended" tables are not recommended by me for one or more of the following reasons: (A) One or more ingredients have been reported to be ineffective or only slightly effective for the product's intended purpose; (B) a more effective product is available; (C) the product advertising or description is likely to heighten consumer expectation beyond actual effectiveness; (D) the product has the potential to cause side effects in the average consumer that are more serious than those generally associated with OTC drugs; (E) the product has the potential to cause serious side effects in persons with specific diseases or disorders; (F) another product is available that is capable of producing the same or nearly the same therapeutic effect without the same risk of side effects; (G) persistent use of the product may cause physical dependency that alters an otherwise normal body function; (H) the product's formulation may reduce the effectiveness of one of its ingredients; (I) this is a multiple-ingredient product that may have no therapeutic advantage over simpler or single-ingredient products; (J) one or more of the product's ingredients may be used for only a short period during the total duration of the illness; (K) the product cannot easily be administered at a dosage level within generally recommended boundaries of optimal therapeutic effect; (L) this is a condition-specific product that is appropriate for use only after a health professional has helped the patient establish a diagnosis.

Hemorrhoids

Any discussion of diseases of the gastrointestinal tract has to end with hemorrhoids.

Hemorrhoids occur in 25 percent of people over age

thirty. Although there are different types of hemorrhoids, you might think of them as varicose veins in the rectum.

The natural habitat of the indigenous North American hemorrhoid can be divided into three areas: the perianal area, the anus, and the rectum. The perianal area is the portion of the skin and buttocks that surrounds the anus. The anus, about $1\frac{1}{2}$ inches in length, is the southernmost portion of the gastrointestinal tract. The rectum is positioned at the end of the large intestine and is separated from the anus by the anorectal line. Hemorrhoids that originate in the rectum (above the anorectal line) are classified as internal hemorrhoids, while those that start in the anus or perianal area are called external hemorrhoids.

So what are hemorrhoids?

As a general rule they are a combination of abnormally large blood vessels and inflamed supporting tissues and skin. In addition to being classified as internal or external, they may also be described as *thrombotic* when the blood vessel has ruptured and formed a blood clot; *cutaneous* when an old thrombotic hemorrhoid has healed and left a skin tag; *prolapsed* when an internal hemorrhoid has protruded beyond the anorectal line; or *strangulated* when the hemorrhoid has grown so long that the anal sphincter muscle chokes it off.

Several factors predispose humans to hemorrhoids. Our upright posture adds the force of gravity to the stresses that are already placed on the rectal blood vessels. Occupations or activities that require prolonged standing, sitting, or muscle strain also contribute. There are even some indications that you can inherit a tendency toward hemorrhoids from your parents.

Precipitating Causes of Hemorrhoids

Abdominal tumors	Pregnancy
Anal infections	Prolonged coughing,
Constipation	sneezing, or vomiting
Diarrhea	Rectal cancer
Heart failure	Strenuous exercise
Liver disease	

Symptoms of hemorrhoids include bleeding, burning, inflammation, itching, pain, and seepage of stool. You should be aware, however, that not all symptoms are present with all types of hemorrhoids. Some are relatively symptom-free, but you should still see a doctor to take care of these hemorrhoids before they start to cause problems.

Nondrug Treatment of Hemorrhoids

The two most important things you can do to help your hemorrhoids are to keep from becoming constipated and to keep your anorectal area clean.

The passage of stool irritates hemorrhoids because of the friction of stool rubbing against the sensitive tissue. Those who allow themselves to become constipated out of fear of rectal pain are in for real torture when they finally do pass stool.

If you have this problem, go back to the section on constipation earlier in this chapter and read about prevention of constipation through proper diet, exercise, and fluids. If you genuinely need a laxative to keep yourself regular, bulk-forming laxatives or softeners are generally recommended for hemorrhoid patients.

Many people find remarkable relief when they use soft tissue and soap and water to wash their bottoms after each bowel movement. Even if you wipe carefully with toilet tissue after a stool, you still leave small particles of feces that keep the hemorrhoid irritated.

Tucks astringent pads are an alternative that you can carry with you when you are away from home. These pads are soaked with witch hazel and do a good cleaning job in addition to relieving the burning sensation.

An occasional sitz bath may also provide relief on bad days. Many pharmacies sell plastic sitz bath pans that conveniently fit over your toilet rim. A proper sitz bath is accomplished by sitting in warm water, about 110 degrees to 115 degrees Fahrenheit, for fifteen minutes. If necessary, you can do this two or three times a day.

Over-the-Counter Remedies for Hemorrhoids

Despite all the hoopla and hype, there is no evidence

that any nonprescription remedy can significantly shorten the course of this ailment. At best, some products provide some relief from some symptoms. Others seem to do nothing at all.

The best advice I can give you is to avoid the temptation to diagnose yourself. If you have rectal pain, itching, or bleeding, go to a doctor. If the doctor diagnoses a hemorrhoid, he or she will advise you on proper treatment. Self-medicating what you *think* is a hemorrhoid can be dangerous business. Don't take chances like that.

Protectants—For Relief from Irritation

For most simple hemorrhoids, the *only* type that you should be self-medicating, a protectant is all you need. Protectants simply protect the hemorrhoid from irritants like sweat, feces, and friction from walking.

There are gobs of protectants on the market. They include cod liver oil, mineral oil, cocoa butter, shark liver oil, and zinc oxide.

Zinc oxide ointment does a pretty good job, but the one that seems to work best is petrolatum, or petroleum jelly—plain old Vaseline. None of the more esoteric or expensive protectants listed above do a better job than zinc oxide or petrolatum. In fact, the petrolatum ointment base in some of these commercial products is probably the most effective ingredient.

Anesthetics—Pain Relief with Possible Side Effects

When topical anesthetics are applied directly to the painful hemorrhoid, they can numb the area and provide relief from the pain, burning, and itching that are so distracting and uncomfortable. Unfortunately, many of them don't work as well as we would like.

Only benzocaine and pramoxine have been found to be both safe and effective for use on hemorrhoids. One of the problems with all topical anesthetics is that the rectal area is a good site for drug absorption, and some topical anesthetics are toxic if absorbed through the skin.

Topical anesthetics can also sensitize the skin, causing

rashes and allergic reactions that can further inflame the hemorrhoidal area. These reactions not only make you more uncomfortable, but can also prolong the healing process.

Topical anesthetics should be used only on painful or itching hemorrhoids, and only after a doctor has examined you. Anesthetic hemorrhoidal ointments provide no more relief than do the protectants for nonpainful hemorrhoids, but they are capable of causing some very uncomfortable rectal rashes.

Astringents—Safe and Effective for Some Cases

Astringents work by coagulating protein in the cells they contact. This causes a "puckering" feeling and reduces some of the inflammation in the affected area.

Astringents are safe and may also be effective in relieving some people's symptoms. I have mentioned two of them previously, zinc oxide and witch hazel. Witch hazel is the active ingredient in Tucks pads.

Calamine is another potentially effective astringent. Much of calamine's efficacy comes from the fact that it contains zinc oxide.

Counter-Irritants—Senseless Remedies

These are the same group of drugs that you rub over a sore muscle for relief of aching pains. I didn't recommend them in the chapter on pain, and I don't recommend them now.

Counter-irritants work by irritating the skin to fool the nerves into interpreting the sensations as cooling or tingling. It just doesn't make much sense to me to put an irritant onto an already inflamed area.

Some of the more common hemorrhoidal counter-irritants include camphor, hydrastis (golden seal), juniper tar, and turpentine. I don't recommend them.

Vasoconstrictors—Of Questionable Value

The vasoconstrictors in hemorrhoidal products work in basically the same way as the nasal decongestants we discussed in chapter 2. They constrict blood vessels, thereby decreasing blood flow into the area and decreasing some of the swelling.

Some people suggest that vasoconstrictors may be used to treat bleeding hemorrhoids. There is no conclusive evidence that they are effective in controlling rectal bleeding, and they may be dangerous if they delay you from getting effective treatment. *Never self-medicate any type of rectal bleeding.* Get your doctor immediately for a professional diagnosis and proper treatment.

Vasoconstrictors are capable of causing some of the same side effects as the nasal decongestants you take for a cold. It makes no sense to expose yourself to additional hazards when it isn't likely that these drugs will help your condition.

Keratolytics—Not Recommended

These are drugs that peel off the outer layer of skin over the hemorrhoid and anything else that gets in the way.

Does this sound smart?

By their very nature these drugs are irritating, which is usually the last thing you want when you have a hemorrhoid. Some products contain keratolytics to clear the way so that other drugs in the preparation can get into the diseased area. This sounds all right until you consider that no drug has ever been proven to resolve hemorrhoids faster than nature itself.

Antiseptics—No Better Than Soap and Water

Using antiseptics in hemorrhoidal products seems like a good idea because they can clear away all the bacteria that live around the rectum and anus, right?

Wrong!

Billions of little bugs live in and around the body's waste disposal system. Even the most effective antiseptic or antibiotic leaves millions of microorganisms in the vicinity of the hemorrhoid.

Antiseptics have not been proven to improve hemorrhoidal healing time, and many products that contain these drugs use them only as preservatives to ensure that the medication itself doesn't get contaminated. In any event, soap and water probably do as good a job of cleaning the anorectal area as the best antiseptic.

Wound-Healing Agents—There Are None

There is no effective wound-healing agent. Period.

Many claims have been made for products containing drugs that supposedly improve wound- or hemorrhoid-healing time, but none have been proven to work. Some of these agents include shark liver oil, skin respiratory factor, cod liver oil, vitamins A and D, and Peruvian balsam.

Products such as Preparation H and A&D ointment are commonly used for hemorrhoids. Despite the presence of "wound-healing" agents in them, they probably derive most if not all of their effectiveness from the fact that they contain petrolatum, a simple protectant, as their ointment base.

Hydrocortisone—No Proof Yet of Effectiveness

The newest OTC entry into the race for your hemorrhoid dollar is hydrocortisone. This is an anti-inflammatory drug that has some potential for relieving some of the itching and swelling that may accompany a hemorrhoid.

Despite the fact that this drug is widely marketed for this purpose, there is surprisingly little research to determine the role of hydrocortisone in OTC concentrations in the treatment of hemorrhoids. OTC doses of hydrocortisone have not, in my opinion, been fully evaluated either for safety or efficacy in treating this condition. Until this investigation is done, I cannot recommend any OTC hydrocortisone product for treatment of hemorrhoids.

Dosage Forms of Hemorrhoidal Products

Once you decide on which hemorrhoidal product you are going to use, the next stumbling block is to determine which dosage form to select. While hemorrhoidal medications are also available as foams and suppositories, the ointments and creams are the most commonly used.

Ointments and creams can be applied with either the "pile pipe" that is included in the box with the ointment tube, or you can use your fingers, which are included in your basic anatomy.

The best way to handle a pile pipe is to lift it carefully out of the box, hold it firmly between your index finger and thumb, walk over to the trash can, and throw it away.

Pile pipes have one advantage: They allow you to insert medication high up into the rectum where your finger cannot reach. However, most OTC's don't work very well up there. If they are used, pile pipes must be flexible and well-lubricated. They can be dangerous because they can cause abrasions, bruises, and even perforations of the rectum. They have too much potential for harm and too little potential for benefit.

The fingers are the best applicators for hemorrhoidal products. For those who question the esthetics of the procedure, rubber gloves or rubber finger coverings can be purchased in most pharmacies.

After ointments and creams, the next most popular dosage form is the suppository. The main advantage of suppositories is that they slowly spread their ingredients over the hemorrhoid as they melt. Their major problem is that it is next to impossible to keep them in the right place.

When a suppository is inserted into the anus it has a tendency to ride up into the rectum and lower colon and get lost. In addition, when something is inserted into the rear end, the natural tendency is to have a bowel movement. If this happens, the whole works ends up in the toilet, where it doesn't do a bit of good.

A more recent innovation has been the introduction of medical foams for rectal use. The foams usually contain the same medication that you can get in an ointment, but the high tech forms cost you more. They have no proven advantage over ointments.

☙

The Pharmacist's Prescription for Hemorrhoids

General Information

Constipation can be a contributing factor to development of hemorrhoids. Prevent constipation by ensuring an adequate intake of dietary fiber and fluids and by getting enough exercise.

Straining with bowel movements often aggravates hemorrhoids. Do not strain with bowel movements and do not sit on the toilet for longer than two minutes at a time.

Recommended Treatment

Cleanse your anus, preferably with soap and water, after each bowel movement. Astringent cleansing pads are suitable alternatives.

If a hemorrhoidal medication is used, apply it *after* a bowel movement rather than before.

Use your gloved finger to apply medication. Do not use a pile pipe.

Sitz baths may be useful in providing temporary relief.

If hemorrhoidal medications are used, use a product that contains a protectant or an astringent.

See Your Doctor if . . .

- You suspect that you may have hemorrhoids or any other anorectal disorder.
- You have any bleeding, seepage of stool, or pain from your rectal area.
- Your hemorrhoidal medication causes pain or causes your condition to worsen.
- You have not gotten relief after seven days of self-medication.

Products Recommended for Hemorrhoids

Astringents
  Mediconet Medical Pad
  Preparation H Cleansing
    pads
  Tucks Cream
  Tucks Ointment
  Anusol
  Tronolane Cream

  Tucks Pads
  Zinc oxide
Anesthetics
  Americaine

Protectants
  Vaseline Pure
    Petroleum Jelly
  White petrolatum

Or the generic equivalent of any of the above

Products Not Recommended for Self-Medication of Hemorrhoids

A & D Ointment (A,I)
Cortef Rectal Itch
    Epinephricaine
    Ointment (I)
Lanacane (I)
Pazo Suppositories (I)
Peterson's Ointment (I)
Pontocaine Ointment (I)
Preparation H Ointment
    (A,I)
Preparation H
    Suppositories (A,I)

Nupercainal Ointment (B)
Nupercainal Suppositories
    (B)
Ointment (B)
Pazo Ointment (I)
Rectal Medicone
    Suppositories (I)
Rectal Medicone Unguent
    (I)
Wyanoid Ointment (I)
Wyanoid Suppositories (I)

Or the generic equivalent of any of the above

The products listed in the "Not Recommended" tables are not recommended by me for one or more of the following reasons: (A) One or more ingredients have been reported to be ineffective or only slightly effective for the product's intended purpose; (B) a more effective product is available; (C) the product advertising or description is likely to heighten consumer expectation beyond actual effectiveness; (D) the product has the potential to cause side effects in the average consumer that are more serious than those generally associated with OTC drugs; (E) the product has the potential to cause serious side effects in persons with specific diseases or disorders; (F) another product is available that is capable of producing the same or nearly the same therapeutic effect without the same risk of side effects; (G) persistent use of the product may cause physical dependency that alters an otherwise normal body function; (H) the product's formulation may reduce the effectiveness of one of its ingredients; (I) this is a multiple-ingredient product that may have no therapeutic advantage over simpler or single-ingredient products; (J) one or more of the product's ingredients may be used for only a short period during the total duration of the illness; (K) the product cannot easily be administered at a dosage level within generally recommended boundaries of optimal therapeutic effect; (L) this is a condition-specific product that is appropriate for use only after a health professional has helped the patient establish a diagnosis.

6

OTC's and Today's Woman

No one is born a woman.
One is merely born a female,
and becomes a woman.
—Simone de Beauvoir
(1908–1986)

A woman's reproductive system is a marvelously complex collection of anatomic structures and physiologic functions that initiates life, nurtures it while it takes human form, protects and provides for it during the birth process, and even feeds it in infancy.

From menarche to menopause, a woman is primed to initiate the life process. Unfortunately, this constant state of readiness, in the form of the menstrual cycle, exacts a heavy toll.

Menstrual Difficulties

Your menstrual cycle has two basic purposes. It causes the release of a mature ovum or egg, and it prepares your uterus for implantation of a fertilized egg. If fertilization doesn't occur, which is usually the case, the flow of hormones stops, the interior lining of the uterus breaks away from its wall, and the menstrual flow begins. A week later, the process starts all over again.

The average menstrual cycle lasts twenty-eight days but may be as short as twenty days or as long as forty-five. The duration of the menstrual flow, or period, is also variable. It can range from two to eight days. During that time most women lose two to three ounces of blood. That amount of blood loss every month, even in women with good diets, can lead to anemia.

Premenstrual Syndrome and Menstrual Cramps

As if the monthly menstrual flow itself were not enough, the majority of women experience either premenstrual syndrome or menstrual cramps. Some have both.

Premenstrual syndrome, or PMS, may affect as many as 90 percent of women. About one-third of women report that they have some degree of mental or physical disability during their bouts of PMS.

Symptoms of Premenstrual Syndrome

Acne	Drowsiness
Anxiety	Fainting
Bloating	Fatigue
Breast tenderness	Headaches, including
Constipation	migraines
Cramps	Hostility
Craving for sweets,	Irritability
especially chocolate	Lack of energy
Crying spells	Lightheadedness
Depression	Mental stress
Disrupted sleep	Mood swings
Dizziness	Swelling in the legs

The most common symptoms of PMS are mental stress, irritability, mood swings, and sometimes abnormal drowsiness. These symptoms may be accompanied by muscle aches, thirst, cravings for sweets or chocolate, and a feeling of bloating.

For most women the symptoms of PMS are relieved with the onset of their periods. The cause of PMS still has not been pinpointed, but it appears that the rapid changes of hormone levels that occur in the last few days before menstruation may trigger the reaction.

Dysmenorrhea, or menstrual cramps, is the second most common gynecologic problem women encounter. At least half of all menstruating women experience at least mild cramping at the onset of their periods. Normally these cramps disappear after a day or two, without causing any significant disruption of activity. However, about 10 percent of women have severe cramping. The cramps may also be associated with nausea, diarrhea, headache, abnormal drowsiness, lack of appetite, and irritability.

Menstrual cramps are usually worst in a woman's late teen years or early twenties. Thereafter they diminish with age. They also lessen after the birth of children. Cramps that start only after a woman is past age twenty suggest that she may have other physical problems, and a visit to the doctor is in order.

One of the most significant advances in the treatment of dysmenorrhea came fairly recently with the discovery of chemicals called prostaglandins in menstrual blood. Prostaglandins are chemical regulators in the body, similar to hormones. The types of prostaglandins that are found in menstrual blood are the same as those that initiate uterine contractions in labor!

This discovery is significant, since we know of several drugs that can control prostaglandins, and through continued research we will surely learn of others.

Treatment for Menstrual Difficulties

In terms of treating menstrual difficulties with prescription or nonprescription drugs, we can treat dysmenorrhea much more effectively than we can PMS. Unfortunately, there is no shortage of OTC products that claim to be effective in controlling PMS symptoms.

Most of the menstrual products on the market contain diuretics, antihistamines, decongestants, or herbs, along with aspirin or acetaminophen. None of them are very effective for PMS, and the analgesic they contain is more effective for menstrual cramps than any of the other symptoms.

A complicating factor in evaluating medications for PMS is that as many as half of all women experiencing symptoms of PMS get better when they are given a placebo. A placebo is a tablet or capsule that contains only inert substances, usually sugar.

Does this mean that PMS is all in your head? That you're

faking these symptoms to get sympathy or extra consideration at home? That you're playing some type of game to get even with the man in your life?

Definitely, absolutely, positively not!

Placebo is one of the most misunderstood medications available. Two research projects at the Mayo Clinic have proven that more than 30 percent of patients got relief from placebo after abdominal surgery. Were these people faking their surgery or their pain? No way!

The high degree of response to placebo in PMS makes it difficult to evaluate OTC drugs that purport to be effective for this syndrome. If you take anything at all for your PMS, you have a 50-50 chance of feeling better. Do you need Midol, Premesyn PMS, or any of the others? Probably not.

If you have problems with PMS, see your gynecologist. The diagnostic procedures and the therapies he or she has available are much more effective than anything available over the counter.

Analgesics—The Best OTC Remedies for Menstrual Cramps

Effective OTC products are available, however, for the treatment of mild dysmenorrhea. The most effective drugs are the same ones we discussed in chapter 3—aspirin, acetaminophen, and ibuprofen.

Since we covered all three in an earlier chapter, I don't need to repeat the information on their uses and side effects. However, there are some things you should know about their specific actions for dysmenorrhea.

Aspirin and acetaminophen have been used for menstrual cramps for years, usually with disappointing results. The problem is that until recently we didn't know how to use them properly.

Both drugs are effective in reducing the effects of the prostaglandins that provoke menstrual cramps. However, they have to be given *before* the uterine levels of prostaglandins get too high. Therefore, in order to be effective, you should start taking them about two days before your period begins.

While they may be effective if started early enough, that doesn't do much good if your period sneaks up on you. Fortunately, you don't have to watch the calendar. Ibuprofen has become the new wonder drug for treatment of cramps. Gynecologists discovered this several years ago when it was available only by prescription as Motrin and Rufen. In 1984 the Food and Drug Administration approved the sale of ibuprofen over the counter.

OTC ibuprofen, sold as Advil and Nuprin, is good news for women with menstrual cramps. Surveys have shown that users get 66 to 100 percent relief with doses of 400 milligrams (two tablets) four times a day. You can start taking the drug when the pain begins; you don't have to anticipate your periods as you do with aspirin.

The only major drawback to ibuprofen is the fact that people who are allergic to aspirin are probably also allergic to ibuprofen. Aspirin-allergic people should *never* take ibuprofen except under a doctor's close supervision. The only alternative for these people is acetaminophen (Datril, Tylenol).

Only two other OTC drugs have been judged by the FDA advisory panel to be safe and effective for the treatment of menstrual cramps. They are the weak antispasmodic cinnamedrine and the antihistamine pyrilamine. Even at that, the FDA panel couldn't establish that cinnamedrine by itself is effective for menstrual cramps. And pyrilamine has all the side effects of the antihistamines, including drowsiness.

Both of these drugs pale in comparison with ibuprofen.

Toxic Shock Syndrome—It Hasn't Disappeared

Many women believe that toxic shock syndrome, or TSS, has disappeared because they no longer hear about it on the evening news. Unfortunately, that isn't the case. TSS is nearly as common now as it ever was.

TSS is an illness that develops rapidly, usually in young, healthy women during or within two days of the end of their menstrual periods. Women between the ages of fifteen and twenty-four are at greater risk than older women. A woman's risk of developing toxic shock is about 1 in 30,000 per year. Until 1981, when effective treatments were discovered, 10 percent of affected women died. In 1981 the FDA reported that the mortality rate from toxic shock was down to 3 percent.

Symptoms of Toxic Shock Syndrome (TSS)

Only a few of the following may be present:

Bleeding	Low blood pressure
Confusion	Muscle pain
Decreased urination	Nausea and vomiting
Diarrhea	Small red spots on the
Difficulty breathing	skin
Disorientation	Sore throat
Easy bruising	Sunburn-like rash that
Fainting	occurs on the palms and
High fever	soles
Irritability	

The warning signs of TSS include sudden onset of fever of 102 degrees Fahrenheit or higher, vomiting, dizziness or fainting when standing up, and/or a rash that looks like a sunburn.

While the overuse of tampons is a definite risk factor for the development of toxic shock, it isn't the only one. About 15 percent of cases of TSS occur either in women who are not menstruating, or in men and boys.

Current medical opinion is that toxic shock syndrome is caused by toxins produced by *Staphylococcus aureus* bacteria. Just how and why these organisms, which normally live on our skin and cause no problems, are able to invade and dump their poisons in us isn't known.

Since the only proven risk factor for toxic shock is the use of tampons, the only advice we can give for prevention revolves around their conservative use. A study conducted by the Centers for Disease Control has shown that TSS is associated with all brands of tampons that have been tested. Their findings indicate that Rely tampons were implicated in 71 percent of cases; Playtex in 19 percent; Tampax, 5 percent; Kotex, 2 percent; and O.B., 2 percent.

Women who wear tampons and have not had TSS seem to be at low risk of developing the problem. However, all women who use tampons should change them at least four to six times per day. It is also thought that alternating tampons with sanitary napkins may be beneficial. Some suggest using tampons only during the day and napkins at night.

Women who have had toxic shock may have as great as a 45 percent risk of developing the illness again. They should not use tampons again unless their doctor has been able to prove that all the staphylococcal organisms have been removed from menstrual and vaginal secretions.

Prevention is the watchword in toxic shock syndrome. TSS can be a devastating, fatal illness that is difficult to treat if not caught early. *If you develop any symptoms of TSS, call your doctor immediately.*

The Pharmacist's Prescription for Menstrual Problems

Self-treatments for premenstrual syndrome are not effective. See your doctor for help.

Mild menstrual cramps can be self-medicated with ibuprofen. Aspirin and acetaminophen are alternative treatments.

To prevent toxic shock syndrome:

Use tampons with minimal absorbancy.

Change tampons at least six times a day during menstrual periods.

Do not use tampons if you ever have had toxic shock syndrome.

See the Doctor if . . .

- You have any changes in the frequency, odor, volume, or appearance of your menstrual discharge.
- You have noticeable swelling before your period.
- Your cramping causes significant pain, limits your activity, or causes you to miss school or work.
- You feel overly tired without apparent reason or have shortness of breath.
- You have vaginal bleeding after menopause or during pregnancy.
- Your cramps do not respond to ibuprofen, aspirin, or acetaminophen.

- Your premenstrual syndrome limits your activities or interferes with interpersonal relationships.

Products Recommended for Treatment of Dysmenorrhea (Menstrual Cramps)

Ibuprofen	Acetaminophen	Aspirin
Advil	Datril	
Doan's	Tylenol	
Ibuprofen Pills		
Haltran		
Medipren		
Midol 200		
Nuprin		
Trendar		

Products Not Recommended for Self-Treatment of PMS or Dysmenorrhea

Aqua-Ban (A,I)
Cardui (I)
Diurex (I)
Diurex-2 (I)
Diurex Long Acting (I)
Humphrey's No. 11 (A,I)
Lydia E. Pinkham
    Tablets (A,I)

Lydia E. Pinkham
    Vegetable Compound
    Liquid (A,I)
Midol (I)
Pamprin (I)
Premesyn PMS (I)
Tri-Aqua (A)

Or the generic equivalent of any of the above

The products listed in the "Not Recommended" tables are not recommended by me for one or more of the following reasons: (A) One or more ingredients have been reported to be ineffective or only slightly effective for the product's intended purpose; (B) a more effective product is available; (C) the product advertising or description is likely to heighten consumer expectation beyond actual effectiveness; (D) the product has the potential to cause side effects in the average consumer that are more serious than those generally associated with OTC drugs; (E) the product has the potential to cause serious side effects in persons with specific diseases or disorders; (F) another product is available that is capable of producing the same or nearly the same therapeutic effect without the same risk of side effects; (G) persistent use of the product may cause physical dependency that alters an otherwise normal body function; (H) the product's formulation may reduce the effectiveness of one of its ingredients; (I) this is a multiple-ingredient product that may have no therapeutic advantage over simpler or single-ingredient products; (J) one or more of the product's ingredients may be useful for only a short period during the total duration of the illness; (K) the product cannot easily be administered at a dosage level within generally recommended boundaries of optimal therapeutic effect; (L) this is a condition-specific product that is appropriate for use only after a health professional has helped the patient establish a diagnosis.

Feminine Hygiene

Americans are obsessed with cleanliness, so much so that
Europeans often complain that all Americans smell like
soap.

Advertisers have recognized this fetish and have created
ad campaigns that have successfully breached woman's last
sanctuary—the vagina itself. Television has convinced
women that the natural secretions of the private parts of their
bodies are offensive to all passersby.

It's this sort of illogic and misinformation that originally
brought us the feminine deodorant sprays. These products
were not only not needed, they caused considerable irritation and uncomfortable rashes in many of the sensitive
areas that were exposed to them.

Douches

Because of side effects, interest in deodorant sprays has
waned, but the new miracle of Madison Avenue is the
douche. Douches come in a variety of colors, odors, and
even flavors. They are available as powders, concentrated
liquids, or in ready-to-use feminine syringes. And they are
seldom, if ever, needed.

What are you trying to wash out with a douche? What
is its purpose? Is it necessary?

In most cases douching removes vaginal secretions,
remnants of menstrual discharge, dead cells from the vaginal walls, and semen. Is it necessary to douche to remove
these wastes?

No!

The vagina is self-cleansing. All of the natural materials
that either originate in or are introduced into the vagina
gravitate outward and are eliminated naturally without help
from any pharmaceutical company. The vaginal wall is
constantly bathed with natural secretions that maintain the
vagina's health and function.

Occasionally women do encounter problems with vaginitis, an irritation characterized by itching and inflammation of the vagina. But self-treatment of itching around the vagina without knowing the cause of the problem could create a serious health hazard. Infections of the vagina, or any other part of your body, can be diagnosed accurately only in a laboratory, not in your bathroom.

Douches may relieve some of the symptoms of an infection, but they can't cure the problem. Some special purpose douches, like Betadine, can be used as an adjunct to your doctor's therapy, but they should not be used for self-treatment. If used improperly, douches may even help to *spread* an infection.

Douches must do something or they wouldn't have been around for so long, right?

True. Douches do serve some purpose. They often make the user feel cleaner and fresher. They also remove odors.

While some physicians say that women should never douche, many gynecologists find that douching does no harm. It just doesn't do much good, either. And you should never douche more often than twice a week.

But if you are going to douche, do it right.

The vaginal tract is sensitive and can be injured easily. Douche bags may be sold with interchangeable douche and enema tips. Accidental interchange of these tips may cause injury or infection. In addition, *douche fluids should be instilled slowly, without excess water pressure*. Ideally, the douche container should not be held or hung more than twenty-four inches above your hips. If you use one of the disposable douches or your own douche bulb or syringe, be sure to use as little pressure as possible.

Interestingly, douches work better if you are lying on your back, rather than sitting on the toilet. The fluid circulates better if you raise your hips and draw your knees up. You'll need to do this in the bathtub or use a bedpan to catch the fluid.

Of course, you'll need to clean your bag, tube, and nozzle carefully after each use. Some recommend boiling the whole works to prevent infection. And you should *never douche if you are pregnant or think you may be.*

Antiseptic Douches—Only if Your Doctor Recommends Them

Some douche products list one or more antiseptics on their labels. The concentrations of most of these chemicals are only high enough to prevent contamination of the product in the bottle. They aren't strong enough to treat or prevent infection.

If you suspect a vaginal infection, you should go to your doctor. While there are some excellent special purpose antiseptic douches on the OTC market, they may not be suitable for use in your case. I don't recommend them unless your doctor approves their use.

Counter-Irritants in Douches—Remedies with No Good Purpose

Are you getting the feeling that some drug manufacturers put counter-irritants in everything? Not even douches are free from these potential irritants.

Some of the more fragrant ingredients, such as eucalyptol, wintergreen oil, and menthol, may cover up odors. However, the "medical" reason for their inclusion in medicinal douches is to relieve itching and to soothe the vagina. While this may sound good, it doesn't make sense. The vagina doesn't have sensory nerves; therefore, nothing can soothe the area and, in fact, you can't feel irritation or itching in the higher parts of the vagina because it lacks this type of nerve fiber.

Acids and Alkalis in Douches—A Slight Difference

Many commercial douche products are "pH adjusted" to alter the natural environment of the vagina. Some are intentionally acidic, while others are alkaline.

It really doesn't make much difference which type you use. Alkaline douches seem to do a little better job of cleaning, but the acid douches are more compatible with the vagina's natural acidic secretions. In either case, the acidity or alkalinity is very mild.

Vinegar Plus Water—A Good Homemade Douche

Many gynecologists feel that Grandma's vinegar and water douche is as good as anything on the market. A simple solution of two tablespoonfuls of vinegar added to a quart of warm water makes a dilute acidic douche.

Besides being cheap and easy to make, a vinegar and water douche also avoids the antiseptics, counter-irritants, and other ingredients that do little good but do have the potential for causing allergic reactions and other side effects. So many women have returned to vinegar and water douches that some companies have started selling them commercially premixed.

The Dangers of Douching

If you feel that you need to douche more frequently than twice a week, you may have a problem that needs your doctor's attention. Most women douche infrequently, if at all.

Be careful of your douching technique. As noted previously, incorrect insertion of douche nozzles can cause injury, and improper cleaning of your equipment may lead to infection.

The more chemicals your douche solution contains, the greater the chance that you will absorb undesirable drugs into your blood and the rest of your body. Obviously, the more ingredients, the greater the chance for side effects. It has been demonstrated that the antiseptic iodine in Betadine douches reaches your blood and eventually goes to your thyroid gland.

Some women use douches as contraceptives. *They don't work in preventing pregnancy.* In fact, if you use a contraceptive foam, suppository, or sponge, *do not douche* for at least eight hours after intercourse. The douche may wash the sperm around the contraceptive and increase your chances of pregnancy.

Speaking of pregnancy, that's the most dangerous time to douche. You are at risk not only of absorbing drugs that can harm your baby, but you can also force deadly air bubbles into the uterine blood vessels.

You are also at greater risk of developing uterine and fetal infections if you douche during pregnancy. The douche fluid can carry bacteria up into the uterus and even up the fallopian tubes.

Under some circumstances douching may be necessary

during pregnancy, but these treatments should be prescribed and monitored by your doctor. Avoid any self-medication during pregnancy.

Interestingly, a group of gynecologists demonstrated that a simple method of bathing was effective in relieving symptoms of vaginitis and was also suitable as a normal cleansing practice. The technique consisted simply of using the fingers and soap in lukewarm water to gently wash the vulva, the anus, and the area between them.

This method seems to be much safer than douching, even if you are only using vinegar and water.

The Pharmacist's Prescription for Feminine Hygiene

General Information
Douching is generally not necessary, as the vagina tends to be self-cleaning.

Recommended Treatment
Cleanse the vaginal and anal areas with mild soap when bathing.

If you feel that you must douche:

> Make a solution of two tablespoonfuls of vinegar in a quart of lukewarm water.
>
> Do not douche more than twice a week, if that often.
>
> Clean your douche equipment before and after each use.
>
> Use proper care in inserting the douche nozzle.
>
> Use minimal pressure when irrigating with the douche fluid.

See the Doctor if . . .
- Your vaginal area has an unusual odor.
- You notice an unusual vaginal discharge.
- You have persistent itching around your vagina.
- You feel that you need to douche frequently.

Recommended Douches
Massengill Vinegar and Water Disposable Douche

Summer's Eve Vinegar and Water Disposable Douche
  Or the generic equivalent of either of the above

Douches Not Recommended for Self-Treatment
  Betadine Douche (L)
  Femidine Douche (L)
  Jeneen (I)
  Massengill Disposable Douche (I)
  Massengill Douche Powder (I)
  Massengill Liquid (I)
  Massengill Medicated Disposable Douche (L)
  Nylmerate II (I)
  Summer's Eve Disposable Douche (I)
  Summer's Eve Medicated Disposable Douche (L)
  Trichotine (I)
  Zonite (I)
  Or the generic equivalent of any of the above

The products listed in the "Not Recommended" tables are not recommended by me for one or more of the following reasons: (A) One or more ingredients have been reported to be ineffective or only slightly effective for the product's intended purpose; (B) a more effective product is available; (C) the product advertising or description is likely to heighten consumer expectation beyond actual effectiveness; (D) the product has the potential to cause side effects in the average consumer that are more serious than those generally associated with OTC drugs; (E) the product has the potential to cause serious side effects in persons with specific diseases or disorders; (F) another product is available that is capable of producing the same or nearly the same therapeutic effect without the same risk of side effects; (G) persistent use of the product may cause physical dependency that alters an otherwise normal body function; (H) the product's formulation may reduce the effectiveness of one of its ingredients; (I) this is a multiple-ingredient product that may have no therapeutic advantage over simpler or single-ingredient products; (J) one or more of the product's ingredients may be useful for only a short period during the total duration of the illness; (K) the product cannot easily be administered at a dosage level within generally recommended boundaries of optimal therapeutic effect; (L) this is a condition-specific product that is appropriate for use only after a health professional has helped the patient establish a diagnosis.

Contraception

All contraceptive methods are designed either to prevent the union of the woman's ovum with the man's sperm or to prevent a fertilized ovum from implanting

Contraceptive Failure Rates

Method	Number of Pregnancies per 100 Women During First Year of Use
Tubal ligation (tube tying)	0.04
Vasectomy	0.15
Oral contraceptives (birth control pills)	4–10
Intrauterine device (IUD)	5
Condom	10
Diaphragm with spermicide	17
Spermicide alone	20
Coitus interruptus (withdrawal)	20–25
Rhythm	20–25
Douche	30
No contraception	80

itself on the uterine wall. Sounds simple, doesn't it? If it were so easy, we wouldn't have so many different kinds of contraceptives.

While several types of contraceptives are available to physicians, only two basic types are available on the OTC market. They are the condoms used by men and various forms of spermicides, or sperm killers, used by women.

While that may not sound like much and while it may look as if nothing works very well, we've come a long way from the time when Cleopatra used crocodile manure and wooden "diaphragms" to prevent conception.

No matter which contraceptive method or product is used, motivation is the key to successful prevention of pregnancy. With the exception of surgery, all contraceptive methods rely on the user to employ them properly and faithfully. To achieve effective contraception, barrier methods and spermicides often have to be pressed into service during heated moments, a factor that contributes to their failure rate.

The ideal contraceptive would be 100 percent effective, free of side effects, cheap, and reversible. There is no such thing.

The selection of a contraceptive method is based on finding the most suitable method for the interested couple. Sometimes some of the effectiveness has to be sacrificed because of side effects or esthetics. The table on page 227 lists failure rates of some types of contraception.

OTC Contraceptives

Nonprescription contraceptives are an attractive alternative for women who are concerned about side effects of oral contraceptives (birth control pills) or IUD's. Unfortunately, the OTC's don't work as well as their prescription counterparts.

Condoms—Among the Most Effective When Properly Used

Condoms, also called prophylactics, protectives, sheaths, or rubbers, are the only form of male contraception available in this country, but they are among the most effective when used properly. However, fewer than 10 percent of couples use this method.

More than 80 percent of condom purchases are made in pharmacies, and women make one-third of these purchases. Condoms have achieved respectability. They are no longer used exclusively by teenagers who slink into a gas station men's room to buy them.

Quality control has also improved. Condoms today are more reliable, break or crack less often than they used to, and are manufactured from a variety of materials.

Genuine lamb skin condoms are the thinnest and most sensitive type, but also the most expensive. Rubber latex condoms are the least costly but may cause allergies or rashes in either a male or female.

Condoms must be used properly to be effective. Since sperm may be present on the tip of the penis well before ejaculation, the condom must be applied before the penis is placed into contact with the vagina or vulva. Some of the better condoms are lubricated for ease of insertion, but you can lubricate the other types if you wish. KY Jelly is a suitable lubricant. Vaseline, petroleum, petroleum jelly, or mineral oil should *not* be used, as they may interact with the rubber in the condom and cause it to break.

When intercourse is ended, the penis should be carefully withdrawn as soon as possible. If you leave the penis in the vagina too long, the condom may slip and sperm can leak out around the open end. Also, you need to hold the open end of the condom firmly against the penis during withdrawal to prevent slippage. Any mistake at this point can negate your earlier caution.

You can also lengthen your odds against pregnancy if the woman uses a spermicide while the man uses a condom. In fact, the effectiveness of the combination of condoms and spermicides approaches that of the oral contraceptives.

Spermicides—A Variety of Choices

The FDA advisory panel on contraceptives has endorsed the use of only three spermicidal agents, and one of them is not commercially available in this country. The other two are nonoxynol-9 and octoxynol-9. At the same time, the FDA panel determined that phenylmercuric acetate and phenylmercuric nitrate were not sufficiently safe and effective for over-the-counter use.

Spermicides do have side effects. Some women and men find them irritating and cannot tolerate their use. Others seem to develop allergies to them. The biggest cause for concern, however, is whether they cause birth defects in the infants that are conceived when contraception fails.

The jury is still out on this one. One small study of 763 babies demonstrated that the risk of birth defects and mental retardation was double that of the general population. A different study that involved more than 5400 babies exposed to spermicides showed that there was no reason for concern.

Since there is no unanimity of opinion in the scientific community over this issue, I suggest that you discuss your contraceptive plans with your doctor before you try any form of contraception.

Spermicides are available in a dazzling array of forms. As you stand at the drugstore's contraceptive counter, should you select a foam, cream, jelly, suppository, or one of the new sponges? All of them do the same basic job—they kill or disable sperm on contact. But they are all used for special purposes that may not be suitable for you.

Creams and jellies. Creams and jellies are intended *for use with diaphragms only.* They provide a protective seal around the edges of the diaphragm so that sperm can't slip around and reach their target.

If you use a diaphragm, your doctor should have explained its use and purpose to you. He or she may have also recommended a specific cream or jelly for your type of diaphragm.

If you don't use a diaphragm, don't use one of these products.

Foams. The foams are the most popular form of spermicide. Most foams come in small aerosol cans with an applicator. Some of the more expensive "convenient-to-use" brands are sold in prefilled applicators. The only advantage to the prefilled types is that they are easier to use if you're in a hurry.

Carefully read all directions provided with your foam before you try to use it. Shake the can well and fill the applicator. Insert the applicator as high in the vagina as you can and push the plunger.

A dose of vaginal foam is only good for about an hour. If more time than that passes, or if you intend to have intercourse again that day or evening, you need to repeat the procedure.

Suppositories. Vaginal spermicidal suppositories are newer and more convenient to use than foams, but some experts feel that they aren't as reliable.

The suppositories are designed to interact with vaginal secretions to produce a foam. The problem is that the manufacturer recommends waiting at least ten minutes for the reaction to take place, and the suppository is only effective for one hour after insertion. That doesn't leave much room for romance and spontaneity.

To make matters worse, one study found that Encare suppositories were still nearly intact fifteen minutes after they were properly inserted in nine out of twenty women examined.

The problems experienced with these suppositories outweigh any convenience they might present.

Sponges. Contraceptive sponges are the newest innovation in the OTC contraceptive market. The sponges are convenient and easy to use and offer one unique advantage—longevity.

The sponges are impregnated (pardon the term) with spermicide and are inserted in the vagina. But unlike the foams and suppositories, the sponge may be left in place for twenty-four hours. In the meantime, you can have intercourse as many times as you like. The sponges also have a ribbon or string attached to the edge to aid removal.

Sponges are expensive, retailing for about $1 each, but the price may be well worth it if the sponge suits your needs. As with any contraceptive, be sure to follow all directions for use carefully.

Douches—Not Suitable for Contraception

There are no effective contraceptive douches.

Folklore tells us that douching immediately after intercourse can prevent pregnancy. Don't believe it! In some areas in the United States, as well as in some underdeveloped countries, the word is that Coca-Cola douches are more effective than any other kind. Don't believe that either! (Although a group of Harvard University researchers did compare the relative efficacy of New Coke, Coke Classic, and Diet Coke as spermicides, they warned against their use for this purpose.)

Douches are ineffective contraceptives for two reasons: First, they can't remove all 250 million sperm released during intercourse—only one has to arrive at its destination; and second, even if they could remove all sperm, you don't have enough time to do it. The first sperm cells show up at the uterine cervix within ninety seconds of ejaculation. You would have to have the douche ready at the bedside for immediate use in order to start it soon enough. And even that is no guarantee of success.

Remember what I said about douching in the section on spermicides? If you use a spermicide and douche within eight hours of intercourse, you run the risk of diluting or washing out your contraceptive protection before all the sperm cells are disabled.

Although douches are still commonly used for contraception, they are a bad idea. There are no ''contraceptive'' douches on the market today.

Withdrawal—Frustratingly Ineffective for Contraception

Coitus interruptus, or withdrawal, is nearly as ineffective as it is frustrating. Withdrawal requires that the penis be removed from the vagina before ejaculation occurs. Unfortunately, millions of sperm can be released before ejaculation begins.

While coitus interruptus is better than nothing, it isn't much better.

Contraceptives Not Recommended for Self-Medication

Anvita (A)	Intercept (B)
Encare (B)	Semicid (B)

Or the generic equivalent of any of the above

The products listed in the ''Not Recommended'' tables are not recommended by me for one or more of the following reasons: (A) One or more ingredients have been reported to be ineffective or only slightly effective for the product's intended purpose; (B) a more effective product is available; (C) the product advertising or description is likely to heighten consumer expectation beyond actual effectiveness; (D) the product has the potential to cause side effects in the average consumer that are more serious than those generally associated with OTC drugs; (E) the product has the potential to cause serious side effects in persons with specific diseases or disorders; (F) another product is available that is capable of producing the same or nearly the same therapeutic effect without the same risk of side effects; (G) persistent use of the product may cause physical dependency that alters an otherwise normal body function; (H) the product's formulation may reduce the effectiveness of one of its ingredients; (I) this is a multiple-ingredient product that may have no therapeutic advantage over simpler or single-ingredient products; (J) one or more of the product's ingredients may be useful for only a short period during the total duration of the illness; (K) the product cannot easily be administered at a dosage level within generally recommended boundaries of optimal therapeutic effect; (L) this is a condition-specific product that is appropriate for use only after a health professional has helped the patient establish a diagnosis.

Choice of a Contraceptive

The choice of a contraceptive method is a highly personal matter. It is beyond my ability to recommend one to you in a book.

Your choice depends on your personal preferences and religious convictions and those of your partner. Other factors include cost, effectiveness, side effects, interference with intercourse, frequency of intercourse, ease of use, and your commitment to regular use.

If you have questions or concerns about the relative merits or disadvantages of the various methods, seek professional help.

Pregnancy

Pregnancy Tests

OTC pregnancy tests are now available for those who are either trying to become pregnant or for those who wonder if their contraceptives worked.

When the do-it-yourself pregnancy test kits became available, many pharmacists and physicians were concerned that pregnant women would delay their initial OB visits and receive suboptimal prenatal care. Fortunately these fears have proved unfounded.

The self-administered pregnancy tests seem to have had a positive impact on prenatal care. Women who aren't sure if they are pregnant can now test themselves at home and then proceed to the doctor if the test is positive. Many women who were reluctant to go to the doctor for a pregnancy test are actually going earlier than they otherwise would have.

The procedure for the test is remarkably simple. You mix a few drops of your urine with the test mixture, which is composed of a solution of specially treated red blood cells from sheep. Add water and let the solution sit.

The specially treated sheep cells seek out human chorionic gonadotrophin, HCG for short. This is a hormone that is produced by the new placenta. If HCG is present, the chances are good that you are pregnant; within two hours the sheep cells will either form a ring or change the color of the solution, depending upon the test used.

Several different types of pregnancy tests are now on the market. Each works a little differently and yields its own distinctive positive and negative response. Brand names of these tests include:

- Advance
- Answer
- Daisy 2

- E.P.T.
- E.P.T. Plus
- Fact

- First Response
- Improved E.P.T.

It is important to study carefully *all* of the directions for use of the particular test you buy and to carry out those instructions precisely.

All of the commercial pregnancy tests are reliable, but they do have limitations. If the test indicates that you are pregnant, there is a 97 percent chance that the test is correct. When you go to the doctor, he or she will probably want to confirm your test result with another test performed in a professional laboratory. This laboratory test is important, since recent pregnancies and some hormonal imbalances can produce false positive results with the OTC tests.

On the other hand, negative test results are only 80 percent accurate with the first test. This 20 percent error rate is usually due to overenthusiasm or worry, whichever the case may be. It's important to wait at least nine days after a missed period before performing the home test. It takes twenty-three days of pregnancy, or an average of nine days after the expected menstrual period, for the normal woman to produce enough HCG to be measured by the test kit.

Negative results after a repeat test are 91 percent accurate. It would be a good idea to call your doctor for advice if your home pregnancy test says you are not pregnant but your period still has not come.

See the Doctor if . . .
- Your pregnancy test indicates that you are pregnant.

- Two pregnancy tests indicate that you are not pregnant, but your period has not started.

Drugs to Avoid During Pregnancy

This section doesn't deal with drugs that you should take for a condition, but with drugs that you should avoid.

More than 200,000 babies with birth defects will be born in the United States this year. This represents about 7 percent of all live births. Nearly half of all children in hospitals are there because of conditions or abnormalities that developed before they were born.

While nowhere near the majority of these problems were caused by drugs taken during pregnancy, we do know that drugs increase the risk of birth defects.

If you exclude iron supplements, which we know are important for the development of the baby, doctors find it medically necessary to prescribe drugs for 82 percent of pregnant women. The average woman takes four drugs during pregnancy, and 4 percent of women take ten drugs. In addition, 65 percent of women take drugs of one kind or other—including OTC's—that were not prescribed by doctors. All of this drug-taking creates definite hazards to your baby's health.

There is very little reliable information on which drugs adversely affect a growing fetus and which do not. Because it would be unconscionable to conduct experiments on drug effects on human babies, we have to draw inferences from animal studies and examine babies whose mothers have taken drugs during pregnancy. Neither alternative is wholly scientifically satisfactory.

The case of thalidomide is a good example of this inadequacy. Thalidomide, the drug that caused grotesque malformations in infants that were exposed to it between 1960 and 1962, doesn't cause birth defects in laboratory animals. For this and other reasons, the drug was used without second thought by many pregnant European women and some Americans. It wasn't until thousands of babies were handicapped that doctors realized thalidomide was the culprit.

While there is a lack of information about the toxic potential of prescription drugs, there is painfully little information on the teratogenic (defect-producing) potential of OTC drugs. *Do not assume that any drug is safe to use during pregnancy.*

But what about the placental barrier? Doesn't that protect the fetus from drugs?

In reality, the placenta acts more like a sieve than a barrier. The placenta strains the mother's blood, filtering out large molecules like proteins and blood cells. Most drug molecules are so small that they slip right through the placenta and pass into the fetus's blood. Rather than hoping that the placenta will shield your baby from the drugs you take, it's much safer to assume that your baby will receive a dose of every medication you allow into your body.

Aspirin

We do know that aspirin has been implicated as a cause of stillbirths, infant deaths, and low birth-weight babies. Aspirin taken in the last days or hours of pregnancy can increase the likelihood of bleeding problems in the newborn. Aspirin may also prolong labor because of its effect on prostaglandins and may increase the mother's blood loss during delivery.

Acetaminophen is considered to be a safe alternative to aspirin in pregnancy, but there are no guarantees.

Alcohol

While there is much debate over the effects of OTC drugs on the unborn, there is good evidence that alcohol, caffeine, and nicotine are harmful to the fetus. Of the three, alcohol is the most harmful.

One of the worst things you can do to your unborn child is to expose it to alcohol. There is no safe level of alcohol consumption in pregnancy; small doses are only less harmful than larger ones.

Women who have one drink per day during pregnancy, an amount many people would consider negligible, give birth to children that weigh less, have smaller heads, and are shorter than babies of women who abstain during pregnancy. Women who have one to two drinks per day during their first three months of pregnancy double their risk of miscarriage. Those who have three or more drinks per day almost quadruple their chances of miscarrying!

Women who drink during pregnancy also increase the chances of their children developing "fetal alcohol syndrome." These children are small at birth, may be mentally retarded, have poor muscle coordination, and are irritable babies. When they grow a little older, half of them develop hyperactivity during their childhood.

The United States Surgeon General has advised pregnant women to abstain completely from alcohol during pregnancy. The Royal College of Psychiatrists in London has made similar recommendations.

The only encouraging news about alcohol in pregnancy is that babies do better if Mom stops drinking.

Caffeine

High caffeine intake has been associated with increased chances of miscarriage. Because of this and the possibility of birth defects, the FDA has removed caffeine from the GRAS (Generally Recognized As Safe) list of ingredients that may be added to foods.

Nevertheless, caffeine is a natural constituent of several foods and beverages, including coffee, tea, cola, and chocolate. Caffeine is also found in a variety of prescription and nonprescription drugs.

If you are pregnant, it would be wise to avoid caffeine or at least limit your consumption.

Nicotine

Women who smoke during pregnancy have a higher than normal rate of miscarriage as well as an increased chance of birth defects.

Nicotine is even more likely than alcohol to produce low birth-weight babies. Makes you wonder about pregnant women who smoke while they drink, doesn't it?

Nicotine seems to do its job without even touching the baby. Studies have shown that only a negligible amount of the drug ever reaches the fetus. However, infrared pictures indicate that cigarette smoking chokes off the blood vessels that supply oxygen and nutrients to the baby. It also reduces the amount of oxygen in the mother's blood, thereby further reducing the amount of oxygen available to the little one.

Breast-Feeding

The hormones progesterone and estrogen prepare the breast for milk production during the last couple of months of pregnancy. As the pregnancy comes to its end, a new hormone, prolactin, dominates the scene. Milk production begins in earnest when prolactin does its job.

The mammary glands in the breast draw nutrients from the mother's blood. These substances include proteins, fats, carbohydrates, vitamins, minerals, and water. Unfortunately, the mammary glands are not highly discriminating. They are not able to distinguish the materials that are supposed to be in the blood from those that are not.

In other words, any substances, including drugs, circulating in a mother's bloodstream may find their way into breast milk and eventually into the baby.

It is safest to assume that any drug, legal or not, that Mom takes can find its way through her milk to her baby. To make matters worse, the baby is more susceptible to drug side effects and toxicities than it will be at any time during the rest of its life.

Very little is known about the effects of nonprescription drugs at this stage of life. No researcher in his right mind would intentionally expose newborn babies to an assortment of drugs for the sole purpose of measuring side effects. Consequently, our present knowledge of these effects is sorely limited.

In addition to drugs that are taken orally, we cannot ignore the potential effects of creams, lotions, and ointments that are applied directly to the breast. Don't put any lotion on your breasts or nipples that isn't intended for use by nursing mothers. The skin around the nipples is sensitive and easily dries and cracks. Masse Cream and lanolin can help relieve these minor irritations, but monitor irritations carefully, because small problems can become serious infections if you allow them to progress.

See your doctor if you are nursing and experience any problems with your breasts.

Analgesics and Breast-Feeding

While we don't know exactly how much is secreted, we do know that significant amounts of aspirin cross from mother's breasts to her baby. We suspect that this may be enough in some susceptible babies to decrease their ability to form normal blood clots.

Based more on what we don't know than on what we do, I advise you not to take aspirin if you are breast-feeding. However, there does not appear to be any problem with acetaminophen (Datril, Tylenol).

Caffeine Consumption and Mother's Milk

About 1 percent of the caffeine ingested by mother finds its way into her milk. This doesn't represent a problem to those who drink caffeine-containing beverages in moderation. However, at least one case of "caffeine jitters" has been reported in a baby whose mother drank large amounts of coffee and cola each day.

Laxatives and Their Side Effects on the Nursing Child

Laxatives like bran and psyllium that aren't absorbed from the intestine appear to be safe to use while breast-feeding. These include the bulk-forming, osmotic, and softening laxatives.

On the other hand, there is some indication that cascara, danthron, aloe, and senna may reach breast milk in concentrations high enough to cause diarrhea and abdominal cramping in the baby.

Avoid Anticholinergics While Breast-Feeding

Various nonprescription drugs contain anticholinergic ingredients that can affect breast-feeding in two important ways. Anticholinergics can cause confusion and psychological disturbances in high doses. They can also cause constipation, flushing of the skin, dry mouth, and difficulty passing urine. These effects could occur in the baby if enough is secreted into the mother's milk. In addition, these drugs are considered to have "drying" effects. Some experts feel that anticholinergics are capable of decreasing production of the milk itself.

Generic names to watch out for include atropine, hyoscyamine, scopolamine, and belladonna. These are found in some OTC sleep aids and diarrhea remedies. Antihistamines also have a mild anticholinergic effect.

There are too many variables to predict the effects of any particular drug on you or your baby. The ability of a drug to affect your baby depends upon the amount of the drug that crosses into breast milk, the amount of milk your baby drinks, the frequency of feeding, and the susceptibility of your baby to any particular drug.

Don't try to figure this out for yourself. Remind your pharmacist or doctor that you are breast-feeding before taking any medication, prescription or nonprescription. They will help you judge the potential benefits of your medication versus the risks to your baby. In some instances it may be necessary to stop breast-feeding, either temporarily or permanently, while taking medication.

Until more is known about the effects of drugs on a suckling infant, which may be never, try to avoid taking any drug that is not absolutely essential to your health.

7

Eye and Ear Problems

All seems infected
that th' infected spy,
As all looks yellow
to the jaundic'd eye
—Alexander Pope (1688–1744)

The eye is truly the mirror of the circulatory and central nervous systems. Many diseases of far-flung areas of the body are reflected in the pupils, blood vessels, and other parts of the eye.

Don't fool around with self-medication for eye problems unless you are *absolutely* sure that the condition involves only the eye. Treating only the ocular manifestations of disease can allow an underlying disease to progress unabated.

Nonprescription ophthalmic drugs don't cure anything; they simply decrease your discomfort until your body corrects the problem. *Infections, burns, and eye injuries should be treated by a doctor, not with OTC drugs.*

People frequently come to the pharmacy for relief of eye problems, only to find that there are no OTC products available for them. Despite pharmacy shelves bulging with numerous and colorful eye, or ophthalmic, products, most of them treat only eye irritations, dry eyes, or are intended for use with contact lenses.

OTC's may provide some relief for itching, stinging, or tired eyes, but don't expect too much from them. Most of the relief they give is short-lived, and they should not be used for more than three days.

Eye Irritation

Conjunctivitis, the proper term for eye irritation, is the most common eye disease in the United States. People with conjunctivitis most often complain of red eyelids, itching and bloodshot eyes, tearing, and, sometimes, sensitivity to light. Vision is not affected by any of these symptoms. Eyes may become irritated because of air pollution, infections, eyestrain, cosmetics, or allergies.

Nonprescription ophthalmic drug products include antipruritics, astringents, decongestants, and antihistamines. Few of these drugs have been proven safe and effective for their intended purposes. Combinations of the same ingredients are equally ineffective.

In general, it is best to identify the cause of the eye problem and then to treat or eliminate it. For instance, if you are allergic to your eye shadow, use a hypoallergenic brand or none at all. If your eyes become irritated when your hay fever kicks up, take care of the hay fever.

In any event, if your eyes don't feel or look better in two days, see your family doctor. If you collect crust or globs of mucus around your eyes, don't even attempt self-medication—see your doctor promptly.

OTC eye drops are intended for treatment of *mild* conditions only, and even then they may not be necessary. For instance, some of these products work well for bloodshot eyes, but if there are no other symptoms, treatment isn't necessary.

Some products are advertised more as cosmetics than drugs. Is it really necessary to "get the red out" of your eyes before an evening on the town?

Precautions to Follow with Eye Medications

The eye can only hold one drop of fluid at a time. Giving yourself two or more drops per dose only wastes medication. If you want to give yourself two or more different eye medications, wait about five minutes between doses. Otherwise the second medication will wash out the first.

Contamination of eye drops is a common problem. These drugs are expensive because their manufacturers take elaborate precautions to ensure that they are sterile when they leave the factory. When you open the dropper bottle you introduce bacteria into the solution. Eye drops contain antiseptics to control this contamination, but the antiseptics can't work forever.

If you touch the tip of the dropper, you may contaminate the solution with more bacteria than the antiseptics can handle. Discard your eye drops if you know that you have contaminated them. It's better to pay for a new bottle than to get an eye infection. It's also wise to throw out any eye drops that have been open for more than three months, even if the expiration date on the side of the bottle has not passed.

Also discard any eye drops that have changed colors or have particles floating in them.

These precautions apply to prescription products as well as to over-the-counter preparations.

Types of OTC Eye Medications

Antipruritics—The Wrong Kind of "Relief"

The most effective antipruritic, or anti-itch, drugs are the local anesthetics. Unfortunately, these are restricted to prescription-only status.

If we need an OTC antipruritic, we have to rely on some of the anesthetics' distant cousins. Antipyrine and our old friends camphor and menthol are included in some products because they have a cooling effect.

Remember how camphor and menthol produce their cooling sensations? They do it by *irritating* the surfaces they are applied to. Is it a good idea to put an irritant in your eye, especially when it's already inflamed? I don't think so.

An additional hazard of antipruritics, and the reason the local anesthetics are available by prescription only, is that they may deaden pain. Pain is one of the body's most effective warning systems. Pain in the eye may be a signal that a foreign body (for example, a splinter, stone chip, or speck of dirt) has taken up residence. Covering up the pain, itching, or irritation caused by a foreign body may delay its removal and result in serious eye injury.

Astringents—Of Doubtful Value

Astringents are supposed to relieve irritation by coagulating proteins on the surface of the eye, but in fact they are of doubtful value.

The FDA advisory panel of eye medications was not impressed with some of the old standby astringents in many products. They included barbarine, hydrastine, peppermint oil, and rose geranium oil.

As a consequence, the makers of one such product, Murine, quietly changed its ingredients but kept the same product name. Murine, which used to contain barbarine, is just one of many examples of products whose present ingredients are very different from what they were a few years ago. Murine now contains a few simple salts that are essentially devoid of direct drug activity. Have you wondered why you can now use it "as often as you like," as its ads state? If it's so mild, does it really do anything for you? Probably not, except as an eyewash.

The only astringent that received the FDA panel's approval was zinc sulfate.

Decongestants—For Occasional Use Only

Many of the ophthalmic decongestants are the same drugs that are used in nose drops and nose sprays. They also have side effects that are similar to those products. But don't use nose drops in your eyes. The eye drops are a different concentration and are specially prepared to be sterile.

Decongestants are effective in relieving simple eye irritation. In fact, the decongestants and zinc sulfate are the only safe and effective OTC drugs available for this purpose. But that doesn't mean that they don't have side effects.

Eye decongestants work by constricting the blood vessels in the eyes. They reduce itching and also "whiten" the eye. But if they are used too often, or doses are given too close together, you can develop a rebound effect in your eye. This is similar to the rebound you can get with nose drops, except that this rebound causes bloodshot eyes instead of a stuffy nose. The rebound is quickly relieved by another dose of decongestant. This sets up a merry-go-round situation where you are continually treating a drug-induced effect with more of the drug that caused the problem in the first place.

Decongestants can also be absorbed through the eye and into the bloodstream, just as the nasal decongestants can be absorbed into the bloodstream through the nose. Consequently, they are capable of causing the same generalized side effects as nose drops. In addition, if you have glaucoma you should not use decongestant eye drops, because they can raise the fluid pressure inside your eye.

If you are going to use a decongestant eye drop to whiten your eyeballs, use them for no more than two days, and don't take them any more frequently than indicated on the package label.

Eyewashes—Soothing When Correctly Used

Products that are designated as eyewashes *cannot* contain active drugs. They are soothing fluids that are supposed to wash dust, pollen, and pollutants out of the eye.

Eyewashes can be refreshing and cooling, but they can also be dangerous if you use an eye cup. If you use an eyewash, *never use an eye cup, even if it comes with the product*. Eye cups harbor bacteria that can enter the eye and cause serious infections.

Instead of using an eye cup, gently drip the solution into the corner of the eye and allow it to flood across the eye surface. Holding the eyelid open and dripping the solution in is usually a two-person operation. Don't try to squirt the solution directly onto the eye. This may cause more discomfort and pain than you started with.

Antihistamines—Best Taken in Tablet Form

If an allergy is irritating your eyes, take an antihistamine by mouth; better yet, call your doctor.

You may get some relief with antihistamine eye drops, but that relief probably results from the fact that these drugs have a mild anesthetic effect. They work not by totally reversing the allergic reaction, but by reducing the sensations of itching and burning. Antihistamine tablets and capsules have been shown to relieve the conjunctivitis that may accompany hay fever.

Anti-infectives—No Suitable Preparations Available

There are no OTC eye drops that can safely and effectively treat eye infections.

Most eye drops contain antiseptics, but they are intended to keep the solution sterile, not to treat infections.

Homemade boric acid solutions are commonly used as antiseptics and eyewashes, but be careful with them. Concentrated boric acid solutions do kill some bacteria, but concentrated solutions also irritate the eye. In addition, you would have to keep your eye submerged in boric acid for at least twenty-four hours for it to have any significant effect.

But what about the boric acid eyewashes that Grandma used to use?

These eyewashes are not only no more effective than any other eyewash, they are also much more dangerous. Boric acid is so toxic that it can be used to poison roaches and other crawling insects. It can also kill people, especially children who play with the crystals or drink the solutions. Boric acid can cause intense, even bloody vomiting and diarrhea, blistering of the skin, fever, seizures, and death.

There is no good reason to have boric acid in your house.

Dry Eyes

As we age we lose the ability to produce tears. By age forty we produce only 50 percent of the volume of tears that we did as teenagers. Those who have serious tear deficiencies, known as dry eye syndrome, complain that they constantly feel as if they have dust in their eyes. They may also experience redness of the eyes and eyelids, burning, and itching. In severe cases they may have open sores on the cornea and conjunctiva.

People with dry eye syndrome have little or no problem during sleep because at that time the eyelid traps moisture on the surface of the eye. The problems begin during the day when this protection is gone and the eye is exposed to drying environmental factors. Wind, dry air, and air pollution do a real number on these people.

"Artificial Tears"—For Temporary Relief of Symptoms Only

Dry eye sufferers often turn first to an over-the-counter eye drop, usually one that is heavily advertised. Unfortunately, these drops often contain decongestants, which cause more dryness. Instead of a decongestant, these people should be using an "artificial tear" product.

The term *artificial tears* is a bit misleading. These solutions don't resemble tears in any way. Instead, they are moisturizers that help to trap the tears that you are able to produce.

Artificial tears can be godsends to many people, but don't use them without medical supervision. If you don't use them properly, or if your dry eye problem has progressed to a serious point, you could be damaging your eyes by delaying proper treatment.

While artificial tears relieve some of the symptoms of dry eyes, *they do nothing to correct the cause.* Do not use artificial tears for longer than three days without checking with your doctor.

You may find that you need to dose yourself with these drops as often as every hour to relieve symptoms. Fortunately, they contain no harmful active drugs. Most of them contain ingredients that form a protective gel over the surface of your eyes. The gel is intended to trap moisture; however, the constant movement of your eyelid over the surface of your eye wears the protection away, making frequent doses necessary. (Take the same precautions when using artificial tears as you would when using other types of eye drops.)

The most common complaint about artificial tear products is that they cause a crust to form in the corners of the eyes. This is just a collection of the gel material and is not a serious problem.

A significant problem, however, may occur when the drops cause pain or blurred vision. If this should happen, stop using the drops and call your family doctor.

How to Give or Take Eye Drops

Here is how to properly take—and give—eye drops, even if you're a coward (most of us resist putting anything in someone else's eyes—even our own child's).

Wash your hands before starting.

Do not touch the dropper with your finger, eyelid, eye, or anything else.

Lie down or tilt your head back.

Using one finger, pull your lower eyelid down to form a pocket.

With the opposite hand, hold the dropper as close to the pocket as you can. *Don't* touch the dropper to the pocket.

Instill one drop into the pocket. Repeat the procedure if you miss the eye.

Close your eye for one or two minutes to allow the medication to spread properly.

Replace the cap on the dropper bottle.

Alternate Procedure

Some people cannot tolerate the sight of a dropper close to the eye. If this is your problem . . .

Close your eye and instill the drop in the corner of the eye closest to the nose.

Slowly open your eyelid to spread the medication across the surface of the eye.

Use the same procedures in administering eye drops to someone else.

The Pharmacist's Prescription for Eye Problems

Do not try to self-medicate any eye condition. Dry eyes, conjunctivitis, and eye infections may all look alike. See your pharmacist or doctor for advice prior to self-treatment.

Never self-medicate if your eye problem has altered your vision.

Do not self-medicate with decongestants if you have glaucoma.

See the Doctor if . . .
- You injure your eye.
- You have pain in the eye.
- You have blurred or altered vision.
- Your eye tears continuously.
- You have a "black eye."
- You have foreign material in your eye.
- You have been taking decongestant eye drops for more than two days or artificial tears for more than three days.

Recommended Eye Solutions

Decongestants or astringents
  Clear Eyes
  Degest 2
  Isopto-Frin
  Murine Plus
  Naphcon
  Visine
  Zincfrin

Artificial tears
  Hypotears
  Isopto Plain
  Liquifilm Forte
  Liquifilm Tears
  Lyteers
  Neo Tears
  Tearisol
  Tears Naturale
  Tears Plus
  Ultra Tears

Eyewashes
  Dacriose
  Eye-Stream
  Murine

    Or the generic equivalent of any of the above

Eye Solutions Not Recommended for Self-Medication

Decongestants or astringents
  Murine (B)
  Prefrin Liquifilm (I)

Eyewashes
  Blinx (F)
  Collyrium (F)
  Trisol Eye Wash (F)
  Or the generic equivalent of any of the above

The products listed in the "Not Recommended" tables are not recommended by me for one or more of the following reasons: (A) One or more ingredients have been reported to be ineffective or only slightly effective for the product's intended purpose; (B) a more effective product is available; (C) the product advertising or description is likely to heighten consumer expectation beyond actual effectiveness; (D) the product has the potential to cause side effects in the average consumer that are more serious than those generally associated with OTC drugs; (E) the product has the potential to cause serious side effects in persons with specific diseases or disorders; (F) another product is available that is capable of producing the same or nearly the same therapeutic effect without the same risk of side effects; (G) persistent use of the product may cause physical dependency that alters an otherwise normal body function; (H) the product's formulation may reduce the effectiveness of one of its ingredients; (I) this is a multiple-ingredient product that may have no therapeutic advantage over simpler or single-ingredient products; (J) one or more of the product's ingredients may be used for only a short period during the total duration of the illness; (K) the product cannot easily be administered at a dosage level within generally recommended boundaries of optimal therapeutic effect; (L) this is a condition-specific product that is appropriate for use only after a health professional has helped the patient establish a diagnosis.

Contact Lenses

Who wears contact lenses? Only vain people who think they don't look good in glasses?

Not at all. The typical contact lense wearer uses them because he or she can see better and because lenses are usually more comfortable and less cumbersome than glasses.

Contrary to popular belief, contact lenses are not a new concept. Contact lens use was first projected as far back as 1888. The first plastic contacts were developed in the United States in 1948, and the first nonexperimental fittings were done in 1955.

Half of all Americans have vision problems that require correction; more than 10 percent of these, or close to 14 million people, wear contact lenses. More than twenty-five laboratories currently produce two basic types and more than thirty brands of lenses. The choice of types and brand of lens appropriate for you is complex and one that only you and your eye doctor can make.

While lenses can provide certain advantages to the wearer, they also pose hazards. No matter how well it is made, a contact lens is still a foreign body, an alien substance, a particle in the eye. If the lens is going to be compatible with the wearer, the eye itself must work right.

The single most important factor in successful contact lens usage is adequate tear production.

Contact lenses are optically molded bits of plastic that float above the surface of the eye. Tears are the vehicle that the lenses float on or in. Any occupation, physical condition, or drug that changes the character of tears or decreases their production can make contact lenses unbearable. Naturally, any person who has frequent eye infections should avoid contacts because the lenses can trap bacteria next to the eye and protect them from the medicinal action of antibiotic eye drops.

Occupations that expose the wearer to airborne dust, dirt, sand, wind, glare, fumes, or extreme cold can cause eye irritations that are aggravated by contacts. Tear production is often reduced during pregnancy and as part of aging. Drugs that reduce tearing include prescription-only diuretics (water pills), oral contraceptives, tranquilizers, and antidepressants. Over-the-counter antihistamines and decongestants can also interfere with proper tearing. The drying effects of these drugs are discussed in chapter 2.

Types of Lenses

Contacts are usually described as being either *hard* or *soft* lenses. Another type of lens, *extended wear,* is actually a soft lens that has been developed for longer wearing time.

Hard Lenses—Their Advantages and Drawbacks

Hard lenses are rigid pieces of plastic that float on a surface of tears. They retain their shape when removed from the eye and can take much more abuse than soft lenses. The term *hard lenses* is a bit of a misnomer. They are only hard relative to soft lenses. Hard lenses are much softer than glass and are easily scratched or chipped if handled improperly. A damaged lens can scratch the eye and has to be replaced.

Hard lenses have been around much longer than the soft ones and have several distinct advantages over soft lenses. Hard lenses are relatively inexpensive and durable. A set of hard lenses typically lasts for about ten years, compared to a few months for extended wear soft lenses. They usually provide clearer vision, less distortion after blinking, are easier to store and clean, and are less susceptible to damage from eye drops.

Of course, they also have their drawbacks. Their rigid design causes more eye irritation than soft lenses, and they have more potential for causing extremely painful scratches on the eye surface. Hard lenses are also harder to fit to the eye, and it takes longer for the eye and inside of the eyelid to adjust to their presence. If all goes well, it takes about two weeks to break in a new pair of hard lenses.

Soft Lenses—Their Advantages and Drawbacks

Soft lenses are thin, highly flexible plastic discs that may be as much as 80 percent water. When placed in the eye, a soft lens molds itself to the contour of the eye. Soft lenses are much more comfortable to wear than hard lenses because they accommodate better to the eye's environment.

Soft lenses must be handled with extreme care when they are removed from the eye. The thickest soft lenses are only one-fifth of a millimeter thick, and nearly half of that is water! They tear easily, and a torn lens is worthless. In addition, they have to be kept in solution at all times. Drying causes them to crinkle like little balls of cellophane, and they become extremely brittle. If you're lucky, you may be able to salvage a dried lens by dousing it in a soaking solution, but you should have your eye doctor check it for damage before putting it back in your eye.

Comfort is the main reason for wearing soft lenses. Because they are less of an intrusion into the eye than are hard lenses, the break-in time for a new user is often less than a week. Depending upon the individual's tolerance for the lenses, soft lenses may be worn for as much as sixteen hours a day, compared to about twelve hours for hard lenses. Extended wear lenses, a variation on soft lenses, can be worn for as long as thirty days without removing them!

Soft lenses also have their disadvantages. It is difficult to correct astigmatism with soft lenses, and cleaning and storage is a nuisance. Their biggest disadvantage, however, is their lack of durability. In addition to tearing easily during removal or insertion, they also absorb mucus and protein from tears. These secretions cause them to cloud and require special cleaning procedures. You should consider yourself lucky if your soft lenses last two years. Extended wear lenses may have to be replaced as often as every six months.

The Importance of Cleaning and Disinfecting Contacts

One of the keys to contact lens care is the proper use of the various solutions. Half of all contact lens problems are due to inadequate cleaning and disinfecting. The solutions are essential to the maintenance of your lenses and must be used religiously. Solutions are labeled for use with either hard or soft lenses. *Never use hard lens solutions for your soft lenses or vice versa.*

Hard Lens Solutions

Hard lenses are easy to care for compared to soft lenses. The four basic hard lens solutions are cleaning solutions, wetting solutions, soaking solutions, and multifunctional solutions.

In addition to their active ingredients, the solutions also contain stabilizers, buffers, and preservatives to extend the useful life of the product. Unfortunately, it is possible for a buffer in one type of solution to react with a preservative in another. These interactions reduce the effectiveness of the solutions and may damage the lens. You can avoid these problems by using solutions that are all made by the same manufacturer. Solution manufacturers take great care to be sure that all of their solutions are chemically compatible with each other.

Cleaning solutions. Tiny glands lining the inside and edge of the eyelids and surface of the eye release their secretions into tears. Unfortunately for your contact lenses, tears are more than just water. They also contain salts, mucus, proteins, enzymes, and particles of trapped dust and dead bacteria. These all congeal to form the slime that we wash out of the corners of our eyes each morning.

When you have plastic lenses in your eyes, some of these materials embed themselves in the plastic. This makes the surface of the lens irregular, and if not removed, clouds and eventually ruins the lens. Cleaning solutions remove this junk.

Hard lenses should be cleaned with a cleaning solution each day. The most common way to do this is to hold one lens between the index finger and thumb, place a drop or two of the solution directly on the lens, and gently rub the solution into the lens with the fingers.

When you've finished cleaning, be sure to rinse the lens thoroughly. Cleaning solutions contain detergents that can irritate the eye if they are not removed before insertion or storage.

Wetting solutions. Since the eyelid has to slide over the surface of the contact lens, the lens has to be made "slick." This is the function of wetting solutions. These solutions lubricate the lens, provide a cushion for the lens to ride on, and consequently protect the lens while it is in the eye.

Use wetting solutions after thorough rinsing. Set the lens on the finger you intend to use for insertion and place a drop of solution into the concave (cuplike) surface of the lens. Hold the lens up to a light to be sure that all surface areas are wet and then place it in the eye.

Some people use saliva as a wetting agent. Don't even think about it! Saliva is loaded with bacteria and can cause ferocious infections. If your lens accidentally pops out away from home, it's better to use a drop of tap water than saliva.

Soaking solutions. When you take your lenses out, clean them with a cleaning solution, rinse with water, then store them in a soaking solution. Soaking solutions keep the lenses moist, inhibit bacteria, and help to remove some of the debris that accumulates on them when they are in the eye.

Never store your lens in tap water or any other solution other than a soaking solution. Water not only can't remove bacteria, it provides a favorable environment for bacterial breeding.

Multifunctional solutions. Wouldn't it be nice if someone would make a single solution that you could use for cleaning, wetting, and storage. The good news is that somebody does. The bad news is that multifunctional solutions don't work as well as the combination of individual solutions.

The problem is that these solutions are a compromise. They just can't work as well as separate solutions. For instance, if they contained as much detergent as cleaning solutions, they would burn your eyes when you used them as wetting solutions.

Multifunctional solutions are convenience items. They are an alternative for people who travel and would prefer to carry one bottle of solution rather than three. They also reduce the clutter on the bathroom vanity.

Try them if you wish. Your eyes will tell you if you made the right decision.

Soft Lens Solutions

Soft lens products are completely different from hard lens solutions. *Never use solutions that are not intended for your type of lenses.* As a general rule, solutions developed for soft lenses may be used for extended wear lenses. However, check with your eye doctor to make sure about your type of lenses. Some products are intended only for use with specific brands of lenses.

As is the case with hard lenses, it is best to buy all of your soft lens solutions from the same manufacturer. Chemical reactions can result from mixing and matching and can damage your lenses. It's a lot safer to pay a little extra for the right solution than to risk ruining your lenses.

Because the characteristics of soft lenses are totally different from those of hard lenses, they require radically different care and handling. Hard lenses tolerate much more abuse than soft lenses. The basic products for soft lenses are cleaning products, rinsing solutions, and disinfecting solutions.

Cleaning products. Cleaning products are of two types—solutions that temporarily remove deposits from the lens, and enzyme tablets that provide more thorough cleaning.

Cleaning solutions are basically wetting agents that dissolve some of the oils that collect on the lens surface and increase the clarity of the lens. These solutions can be used as stopgaps between enzyme treatments or in addition to enzymatic cleaning. Cleaning solutions should be completely rinsed off with saline solution before inserting the lens in the eye, because they can cause intense irritation.

Enzymes are the primary means for removing protein and mucus deposits from soft lenses. Proteins begin to form noticeable deposits in as little as seven days. Once these proteins become tightly bound to the plastic in the lens, there is little you can do to remove them.

Papain, the same enzyme used in meat tenderizers, is the most common contact lens enzyme. Because the enzyme is not stable in solution for very long, papain is sold as tablets in foil packets. Product directions instruct you on how to make your enzyme solution properly with distilled water or saline.

You should soak your soft lenses in the enzyme solution for at least four hours every week. Rinse them thoroughly with saline when you remove them from the solution.

Extended wear lenses are a slightly different story. These lenses have a much greater water content than regular soft lenses. Consequently, the enzyme permeates the lens, latching onto the plastic and refusing to leave when rinsed. Enzyme-embedded lenses cause eye irritation and inflammation when placed back in the eye.

Unless advised otherwise by your doctor, don't soak extended wear lenses for more than fifteen minutes. This is barely enough to remove some of the protein and is the main reason these lenses wear out faster than soft lenses.

Rinsing solutions. Rinsing solutions are simply dilute salt (saline) solutions with preservatives to inhibit bacterial contamination. Rinsing solutions are used between steps of the cleaning process and also to moisten the lens before putting it back in the eye.

These products are also used during the heat sterilization process. All contact lenses need to be kept clean and as free of bacteria, viruses, and fungi as possible. One way of doing this with soft lenses is by boiling the lenses for fifteen minutes.

Heat sterilization requires that the lenses be placed in a special heat unit and submerged in saline solution. However, you must observe two cautions with heat sterilization. First, the lenses have to be cleaned with enzyme *before* the heat treatment or else you can bake the protein deposits onto your lenses and ruin them. Second, make sure your lenses don't dry out during sterilization. Toasted lenses aren't any good to anybody.

If some is good, is more better? Why not sterilize your lenses every day?

Heat sterilization is hard on your lenses. Daily boiling causes deterioration and reduces their effectiveness.

Disinfecting solutions. An alternate method of sterilizing soft lenses is the so-called "cold" or "chemical" disinfection. This method is similar to the soaking solutions used with hard lenses. Like heat sterilization, cold sterilization is done weekly for a minimum of four hours per treatment.

Cold sterilization is initially cheaper than heat sterilization because you avoid the cost of the heat sterilizing unit. Over time, however, heat sterilization is more economical.

Preservatives in Contact Solutions—Caution!

One of the most common difficulties people have with contact lens solutions is sensitivity to preservatives. Preservatives are necessary to prevent contamination of the lens solutions. Those who are completely unable to tolerate preservatives may be able to use expensive preservative-free aerosols.

While there are several preservatives commonly used (benzalkonium, chlorhexidine, chlorobutanol, phenylmercuric nitrate, sodium edetate, sorbic acid, and thiomerosal), the most frequent troublemaker is thiomerosal. If your lenses or solutions irritate your eyes, go back to your eye doctor and try to determine the problem. If you can figure out which ingredient is causing your problem, buy products that use different ingredients. Don't try to tough it out. The solution to the problem is often quite easy.

The Pharmacist's Prescription for Contact Lens Care

Much of the care of contact lenses is simply common sense. The following do's and don'ts make wearing contact lenses a safer and more pleasurable experience.

Do . . .

Follow your eye doctor's directions carefully.

Report to your doctor any eye irritation that lasts for more than a few hours.

Store your lenses only in containers intended for contact lenses.

Wash your hands before handling your lenses. Lenses pick up bacteria and oils from your skin.

Close the drain if you handle your lenses over the sink.

Apply cosmetics, hair spray, and aerosol deodorants *before* inserting your lenses.

Remove your lenses before swimming. Water can wash them off your eyes.

Make sure all your lens solutions are made by the same company.

Remove your lenses if you are going to be working with volatile solvents or cleaning fluids. Your lenses can trap these chemical fumes in your eye.

Check expiration dates and get rid of any solution that is too old. Throw out any solution that has changed color.

Store your lenses only in solutions intended for that purpose. Never use tap water for storage.

Change your soaking solutions daily.

Clean soft lenses *before* heat sterilization.

Make sure solutions for your soft lenses are compatible with your brand of lenses. (This information is usually listed on the side of the solution box.)

Handle soft lenses with particular care. They are easily cut or torn.

Don't . . .

Don't take short-cuts with your eye care. It isn't worth it.

Don't put any medication in your eye while wearing your lenses. Ask your doctor or pharmacist how long to keep your lenses out after using eye drops or ointments.

Don't mix your lenses; they are fitted differently for each eye. Hard lenses may be marked but soft lenses are not. To avoid confusion between left and right lenses, get into the habit of always working with the same lens first.

Don't wear your lenses if your eyes hurt. Inserting contacts into a sore eye usually makes the eye worse. Call your eye doctor if you are having problems.

Don't wear your lenses while sleeping; they reduce the amount of oxygen that gets to your eyes and can result in local ulcers. Only extended wear lenses are designed to be worn while sleeping.

Don't wet your lenses with saliva. You run the risk of serious infection.

Don't rub your eyes while your lenses are in place.

Common Ear Problems

The ear is comprised of three parts: the external ear, middle ear, and inner ear. The tympanic membrane, or eardrum, separates the external from the middle ear. Because the tympanic membrane is a physical barrier, ear drops can only penetrate as far as the membrane will allow. Ear drops, therefore, can only be used to treat disorders in the external ear.

Nonprescription ear drops are more limited than that. OTC ear drops are available for only two purposes—prevention of swimmer's ear and removal of earwax.

Swimmer's Ear

Swimmer's ear is an infection of the external ear canal that may occur when water washes away the protective earwax and allows bacteria or fungi to infect the lining of the ear. This condition can be incapacitating to professional swimmers and divers and is usually associated with swimming in unchlorinated water.

Swimmer's ear is much easier to prevent than it is to treat. Those who are prone to this condition should use protective ear plugs to keep water out of the ear canal, and they should also use drying agents when they come out of the water. Three of the best OTC drying agents are plain ethyl alcohol, isopropyl alcohol, and glycerin. Simply place several drops in each ear canal, let it gurgle down the channel for a minute or two, and then go about your business.

Unfortunately, none of these drugs works very well once an infection has gotten started. If you develop a full-blown case of swimmer's ear, you need to get to a doctor for an antibiotic.

By the way, forget about sweet oil. Some people believe that a few doses of sweet oil can cure ear infections or relieve ear pain.

Baloney!

Sweet oil is nothing more than olive oil. If you treat an ear infection with olive oil, it's likely that the bacteria will thank you for feeding them. *Never put sweet oil into an infected ear.* Sweet oil can help soften hard earwax, but that's all. You can put your olive oil to much better use in your spaghetti sauce.

Earwax

The best thing to do with earwax is to leave it alone.

Cerumen, earwax's proper name, protects the skin in the external ear canal from bacteria. Cerumen also functions as a lubricant and cleanser inside the ear.

Most people think that cerumen is some kind of enemy that has to be eradicated. It's as important to recognize what cerumen does not do as it is to understand what it does.

- Cerumen *does not* cause deafness.
- Cerumen accumulation *does not* indicate that a person is unclean or dirty.
- Cerumen *does not* have to be removed in most cases.

A few people do accumulate more than a normal amount of cerumen. My son is a good example of that. But for most of us, it's more harmful to remove the stuff than it is to leave it alone.

Most people lose their old cerumen without doing anything about it. Cerumen is formed by glands located along the course of the external ear canal. As we move our jaws—by eating or talking, for instance—the ear canal vibrates and moves the cerumen toward the outside of the ear. As it moves it traps bacteria and dust and carries them with it. When it reaches the outside of the ear we can clean it off with a damp cloth, which most of us do each morning.

Earwax is your friend. Contrary to popular opinion, it keeps your ears clean and healthy. We would have constant ear infections without it.

Over-the-counter products are available for those who have excessive earwax. Some products, such as mineral oil or glycerin, can soften wax. This by itself is satisfactory for most people. Dilute solutions of hydrogen peroxide and carbamide peroxide not only soften the wax, but also liquify it.

I don't recommend hydrogen peroxide for this purpose because it can irritate the ear canal if it is not properly diluted, but I have had good results with carbamide peroxide. Just put a few drops in the affected ear and let it do its job.

It you have a serious problem with cerumen accumulation, you may need to use an ear syringe after the ear drops. The ear syringe is a bulb that allows you to force lukewarm water down into the ear canal. The water irrigates the canal and washes out the softened wax.

Ear syringes may be hazardous, however. Don't attempt to irrigate your ear or anyone else's ear unless a health professional gives you complete instructions.

How to Give or Take Ear Drops

Wash hands before starting. Do not touch the tube portion of the dropper with your finger, ear, or anything else.

Lie down with the affected ear up.

Gently squeeze the recommended number of drops into the ear canal.

Gently pull the earlobe back and forth to allow the drops to spread down the ear canal.

Keep the ear in the same position for a few minutes to allow the drops to penetrate.

Some people try to clean their ears with Q-Tips or other cotton swabs, but ear specialists advise against this practice. Ear swabs make better ramrods than cleaners. People who use them aggressively push wax farther down in the ear canal, compacting it against the eardrum. This can cause pain, infection, or hearing loss that requires a doctor's care.

ᛃ

The Pharmacist's Prescription for Earwax

Do not treat earwax unless it is causing a problem.

Do not use ear drops if the ear canal is red or painful.

Fill one ear with several drops of carbamide peroxide and let it sit for five minutes. Turn the head over and repeat if both ears are affected.

Clean the external ear daily with soap and water and a soft washcloth.

If earwax is still a problem, ask your pharmacist or doctor about using an ear syringe.

See the Doctor if . . .
- You have pain in or around the ear or down the neck.
- You have fluid coming from your ear.
- You have hearing loss.
- Your symptoms continue after a course of self-medication.
- Your ear drops cause pain.

Ear Drops Recommended for Softening Earwax
Auro Ear Drops   Dent's Ear Wax Drops
Debrox Drops   Ear Drops by Murine
    Or the generic equivalent of any of the above

Products Not Recommended for Self-Treatment of Earwax
Kerid Ear Drops (K)   Pfeiffer Ear Drops (I)
Oil for Ear Use (I)   Sweet oil (E)
    Or the generic equivalent of any of the above

The products listed in the ''Not Recommended'' tables are not recommended by me for one or more of the following reasons: (A) One or more ingredients have been reported to be ineffective or only slightly effective for the product's intended purpose; (B) a more effective product is available; (C) the product advertising or description is likely to heighten consumer expectation beyond actual effectiveness; (D) the product has the potential to cause side effects in the average consumer that are more serious than those generally associated with OTC drugs; (E) the product has the potential to cause serious side effects in persons with specific diseases or disorders; (F) another product is available that is capable of producing the same or nearly the same therapeutic effect without the same risk of side effects; (G) persistent use of the product may cause physical dependency that alters an otherwise normal body function; (H) the product's formulation may reduce the effectiveness of one of its ingredients; (I) this is a multiple-ingredient product that may have no therapeutic advantage over simpler or single-ingredient products; (J) one or more of the product's ingredients may be used for only a short period during the total duration of the illness; (K) the product cannot easily be administered at a dosage level within generally recommended boundaries of optimal therapeutic effect; (L) this is a condition-specific product that is appropriate for use only after a health professional has helped the patient establish a diagnosis.

8

Losing Weight Sensibly

If you wish to get thinner,
diminish your dinner.
—Henry Sambrooke Leigh
(1837–1883)

How much can you eat without gaining weight?

In most cases, not as much as you would like. There are two basic factors that control your weight: your caloric intake and your metabolism.

Your metabolic rate determines the speed with which your body burns the calories you eat. If you are active and have a high rate of metabolism, you use calories at a faster rate than people who are sedentary and burn calories slowly.

Metabolism is also affected by your sex and age. The average twenty-five-year-old, 150-pound, five-foot ten-inch male burns about 3200 calories per day, but by age sixty-five he burns only 2550 calories daily. By comparison, a twenty-five-year-old, 125-pound, five-foot four-inch woman burns 2300 calories per day, but reduces that amount to only 1800 calories by age sixty-five.

The formula gets more complex with the amount and type of exercise you get in a day. A manual worker may require 1500 calories more than a person of similar age and size with a sedentary job.

While she is pregnant, a woman burns about 300 more calories per day than she does when she isn't pregnant. This rate jumps significantly if she breast-feeds after delivery. The process of milk production takes about 1000 calories daily. This is why many women lose the weight gained during pregnancy faster if they breast-feed.

As long as your daily intake of calories matches your daily

expenditure, your weight does not change. If you burn calories faster than you replace them, you lose weight. The problem for most of us is that we tend to gobble up more calories than we can use. That's when our belts seem to shrink.

When do you decide that it's time to lose weight?

Is it when the Big and Tall Shop can't fit you anymore?

Is it when your body ripples when you walk, but the ripples aren't muscles?

Experts tell us that the average person is overweight when his body weight surpasses his "ideal" weight by 20 percent.

So how can you determine what your ideal weight should be?

We've all seen and compared ourselves to the insurance company tables. Even when I was an anorectic-looking high school kid, these tables indicated that I was borderline fat. How reliable are they?

There are two problems with the insurance company tables. The first is that they don't account for body muscle. Every trim, well-trained, and well-muscled athlete is "overweight" according to the tables.

The other problem occurs because the reprints of these tables seldom give full instructions. They tell you to compare your height with your body build (small, medium, or large frame). They usually *don't* tell you that they assume that you are wearing shoes when you measure your height. Therefore, depending upon the table being used, a man should add one inch to his true height and a woman should add one to two inches. Some tables assume that you weigh yourself nude, while others assume that you are fully dressed. The U.S. Department of Agriculture provides the guidelines indicated in the table on page 266.

An alternate, although also imperfect, method of determining your ideal body weight is suggested by the American Dietetic Association. A five-foot woman with a medium frame should weigh 100 pounds. Add 5 pounds for each additional inch of height. The ideal weight for a five-foot man with a medium frame is 106 pounds, adding 6 pounds for each additional inch. Men and women with small frames should deduct 10 percent from their calculated ideal weight, and those with large frames should add 10 percent.

Approximate Weight Matched to Height

Men		Women	
Height in Inches (barefoot)	Weight Range in Pounds (nude)	Height in Inches (barefoot)	Weight Range in Pounds (nude)
63	118–141	60	100–118
64	122–145	61	104–121
65	126–149	62	107–125
66	130–155	63	110–128
67	134–161	64	113–132
68	139–166	65	116–135
69	143–170	66	120–139
70	147–174	67	123–142
71	150–178	68	126–146
72	154–183	69	130–151
73	158–188	70	133–156
74	162–192	71	137–161
75	165–195	72	141–166

Most people just guess at their body frame—and give themselves the benefit of the doubt. You can use the table below to *estimate* your frame. If you're really obsessed with the need to know your body frame size, you can go to the doctor, get an expensive series of X rays, and have a radiologist give you the verdict.

Estimating Your Body Frame Size

Place a caliper or your fingers on the two protruding bones on each side of your elbow. Measure this distance on a ruler. Compare this measurement with those given below.

This table indicates the measurements for a *medium* frame. If your measurements are less, consider yourself to have a small frame. Larger measurements indicate a large frame.

Height in Inches (barefoot)	Elbow Bone Width (in inches)
Men	
61–62	2½–2⅞
63–66	2⅝–2⅞
67–70	2¾–3
71–74	2¾–3⅛
75	2⅞–3¼
Women	
57–62	2¼–2½
63–70	2⅜–2⅝
71	2½–2¾

Neither charts nor calculations can accurately determine every individual's ideal body weight; they can only provide general guidelines. If you need precise information, you would be better off seeing your doctor or going to a registered dietitian for a nutritional assessment.

Some estimate that between 25 and 45 percent of adult Americans are overweight. The incidence in children may be as high as 15 percent.

So we're a little overweight. Does it really make much difference?

Those who weigh too much are well aware of the social embarrassment, the lack of mobility, and the lassitude that accompanies their condition. Unfortunately, the bad news doesn't stop there.

Men who are 20 percent or more above their ideal body weight double their risk of sudden death from heart attacks. Obesity increases risk of complications during pregnancy and during any type of surgery in men and women.

But there is still some good news, even if you have complications from excessive weight. Many of these conditions improve significantly if you shed some pounds. For instance, obesity overtakes your body's ability to secrete sufficient amounts of insulin. A return to normal weight relieves much of this problem in some diabetics and improves their blood sugar control.

The Complications of Obesity

Accumulation of carbon dioxide in the blood
Arthritis
Boils
Coronary artery disease
Diabetes
Fungal infections
Gallstones
High blood pressure

Hormone imbalances
Kidney disease
Respiratory system stress
Skin ulcers
Stroke
Vaginal itching
Varicose veins
Yeast infections

Why do we gain too much weight for our own good? Many theories try to explain this, but none are proven. However, we do know some factors that influence body weight.

We've already mentioned daily caloric needs and metabolism. It also stands to reason that your body type and lifestyle dictate some of your caloric needs. For instance, a brawny bricklayer needs more fuel to maintain his body than does a computer programmer.

In addition, the longer you have been overweight, the more trouble you'll have losing some of it. If you have dieted in the past and quickly regained your lost weight, your prospects for success this time aren't too hot.

On the other hand, if you gained weight quickly because of disease or medical treatment, your chances of getting back to normal weight are good. That is, they are good if you can control your disease or can discontinue the treatment that caused the weight gain. In any event, be sure to discuss this with your doctor before you take matters into your own hands.

The more weight you carry, the more difficult it will be to achieve your weight goal. The problem is not that a proper weight reduction program will not work, but that you may give up too soon.

Many people fail on weight reduction programs because of inappropriate expectations. Since a strict diet makes them feel miserable all day long, they expect to see progress each time they step on the bathroom scale. It doesn't happen that way. Instead, we tend to lose weight in a stair-step fashion, with periods of small weight reduction followed by periods when we either lose no weight or actually gain some back.

Organizing Your Weight Loss Program

The key to losing weight is not just dieting. You have to combine a sensible diet with regular aerobic exercise. And that's a lot easier said than done.

In order to lose one pound of fat you have to burn off 3500 more calories than you take in. If you intend to diet without increasing your daily activity level, you would have to cut out 500 calories each day to lose one pound per week, and you probably won't lose much fat.

That's a lot of dieting for such a small gain—or in this case, loss. That's why people who want to lose a large amount of weight seldom do.

But there's an easier way. Let your exercise do some of the work for you.

If you walk briskly for twenty minutes you'll burn off about 100 calories. Now you only have to reduce your regular calorie intake by 400 per day to lose a pound a week.

Somehow that doesn't sound too exciting either.

Fortunately, the story doesn't end there. If you faithfully walk at a brisk pace for an hour a day, you'll burn off a considerable number of calories during your exercise. But better than that, you'll also increase your body's metabolic rate throughout the day and even during the night. Regular exercise forces your body to burn calories even when you sleep!

Isn't that better than starving yourself?

Once you get into the habit of regular exercise, stay with it. Consistent exercise not only causes you to lose weight, it also helps you to maintain your desired weight. And you don't have to starve!

Many people can't afford to take an hour out of each day. If this is your problem, you might consider exercising more strenuously for shorter periods. Fifteen minutes of jogging, for instance, is roughly equivalent to an hour of fast walking.

Another alternative is to walk for a half hour in the morning and again before you eat dinner. Exercising before a meal usually has an appetite suppressing effect. Take advantage of any help you can get.

Yet another alternative is to exercise during your regular television viewing time. You can watch "Dynasty" just as well from a stationary bicycle as you can munching potato chips on the sofa.

While you should still limit what you put in your mouth, you don't have to risk destroying your nutritional balance with faddish or overly restrictive diets.

As a safeguard, I recommend that you also take a general purpose multivitamin while you diet. *You should also consult your doctor before starting any diet or exercise program.*

Drugs for Weight Loss

Wouldn't it be easier to just pop a pill to lose weight?

American pharmaceutical manufacturers hope you'll feel that way. Last year they sold $200 million worth of OTC diet aids. But if you bought any of these products, did the manufacturers tell you that they don't work for long, if they work at all?

Over-the-Counter Stimulants

Most nonprescription diet products contain a stimulant as the primary ingredient. Stimulant drugs can increase your energy level while simultaneously decreasing your appetite. Stimulants don't burn calories off of you, but they may make you feel more active and thereby prompt you to be more physically active than you ordinarily would be.

The problem with OTC weight reduction products is that they can't use any of the superstimulants. Because those drugs have too great a potential for abuse, they are limited to prescription-only status.

OTC products have to settle for the second-rate stimulants. The OTC's are limited to decongestants and caffeine.

The use of nonprescription stimulants has two major drawbacks: They don't work very well and they don't work for very long.

Decongestants—The Unfortunate Phenylpropanolamine Bandwagon

When we think of stimulant drugs, most of us tend to think of amphetamine and some of the other heavy hitters. These drugs have been proven to diminish appetite for a few weeks, but they also make many people feel as if they are crawling the walls.

But are decongestants stimulants?

Technically, yes. But they aren't in the same league as amphetamine.

Decongestants, particularly phenylpropanolamine, do have some stimulant qualities. They also cause loss of appetite as a side effect for some people who take them for colds.

But can a product like this be milked for $200 million in sales annually? Apparently so.

To the shock and dismay of many in the pharmaceutical and medical communities, the FDA advisory panel proclaimed that phenylpropanolamine, sometimes abbreviated PPA on product labels, was safe and effective as a diet aid. Phenylpropanolamine was declared to be ''safe'' despite the fact that it is commonly abused. It was said to be effective even though only 25 percent of people who use the drug lose weight. It is supposedly effective even though it has no effect on long-term weight control.

This is absurd!

In the meantime, pharmaceutical manufacturers were ecstatic at the news. They immediately boosted their advertising budgets for diet products, and sales soared. Some manufacturers jumped on the bandwagon by reformulating products so that they would conform to the FDA panel's guidelines.

Unfortunately, as corporate sales figures and profits rose, so did the number of cases of drug toxicity.

The side effects of the decongestants are described in chapter 2. People who are already overweight and those who are anorectic and trying to lose still more weight are particularly susceptible to the effects of phenylpropanolamine on the heart and blood vessels. Fortunately, phenylpropanolamine is the only decongestant approved by the FDA advisory panel for OTC diet aids.

Caffeine—Pointless for Weight Loss

Many products that include phenylpropanolamine also contain caffeine as a second stimulant.

Caffeine shares some properties with phenylpropanolamine. Both drugs cause side effects such as nervousness, anxiety, and irritability. The combination of the two heightens these effects.

Caffeine does not suppress appetite, but it does have a weak diuretic effect. In other words, it causes you to lose water through urination.

Any weight loss caused by urination is short-lived. As soon as you drink a glass of water, you negate the effect of the caffeine.

If anyone knows why caffeine belongs in weight reduction products, please tell me.

The Improper Use of Weight-Loss Drugs

So what if weight reduction products don't work? Is there any real harm in them?

You bet there is!

The following case was reported by Dr. Jeffrey Hyams and his associates in the March 15, 1985, issue of the *Journal of the American Medical Association:*

A 16-year-old girl arrived at the hospital emergency room with dangerously elevated blood pressure and convulsions. She denied using any prescription, nonprescription, or street drugs. The medical team decided to admit her for observation.

On her second day in the hospital her blood pressure rose abruptly, she had a convulsion, and her heart stopped. She was revived and placed on medications to prevent and control convulsions.

Laboratory tests for tumors and other anomalies were negative. For three months her blood pressure fluctuated wildly. She also developed side effects to her medications and some of them had to be discontinued.

Finally, a urine test showed an amphetamine-like compound that was later positively identified as phenylpropanolamine. For unknown reasons, previous urine tests had not shown this result.

She was discharged from the hospital after being advised not to indulge in any substance that contained phenylpropanolamine. She did not have a recurrence of any of her symptoms for a year after discharge.

Kiddie Dope!

Kiddie Dope is the term often applied to stimulant drugs that mimic the effects of amphetamine. Unfortunately, the drugs used in kiddie dope preparations are legal over-the-counter substances. And that's why it's impossible to get rid of them with our current drug laws.

These products usually contain a combination of caffeine, phenylpropanolamine, phenylephrine, ephedrine, or pseudoephedrine. All are legal OTC drugs.

The people who push these drugs on kids don't need to hang around school yards of alleys. They openly advertise in newspapers and youth-oriented magazines! And we can't do a thing about it as long as they do not use deception to sell them.

These drugs are supposed to supply energy and a pleasant high. Sometimes they cause hospitalizations like the one described above. All too often they kill kids.

Nonstimulant Weight-Loss "Aids"

Benzocaine—A Poor Weight-Loss Choice

Local anesthetics were first incorporated into diet products in the late 1950s. The anesthetics, similar to the Novocaine your dentist may use, deaden nerve fibers, including those in the taste buds. The theory is that the anesthetics will dull your sense of taste and diminish your appetite. Benzocaine is the most frequently used drug of this type.

Unfortunately, the numbing sensation in the mouth only lasts for a few minutes. This is the major limiting factor when these same local anesthetics are used in lozenges to treat sore throats. Also, there is no indication that dulling your tastes reduces your appetite.

Some manufacturers use benzocaine in a particularly creative way, putting the benzocaine in a tablet or capsule. Some examples are Caltrim Diet Plan Capsules and Diet-Trim Tablets. When they do this, the benzocaine takes the express route to the tummy and never touches your taste buds. Benzocaine can't numb taste buds if it never touches them.

Local anesthetics can also cause serious side effects. Lidocaine, an anesthetic similar to benzocaine, is known to deaden the throat if taken prior to eating. This can lead to choking and possible asphyxiation.

We normally warn people to avoid eating for at least two hours if they use an anesthetic gargle for sore throats or mouth ulcers. Doesn't it seem dangerous to chew benzocaine gum just before eating?

Bulk-Forming Laxatives—Ineffective Fillers

Are these the same drugs we discussed in the sections on constipation and diarrhea?

They certainly are.

Do they work as well for weight reduction as they do for constipation?

No, they do not.

Then why are they used?

Because the theory sounds good.

When you take a bulk-forming laxative and then drink a glass of water, the drug swells up in the stomach and makes you feel full. The rationale for using these drugs is that you will feel so full from the laxative that you won't want to eat.

It sounds pretty good, but it doesn't work. You do get this stuffed feeling, but studies have shown that the laxative moves out of the stomach and down into the intestine in as little as a half hour. Then you get hungry again.

Another problem with these drugs is that they don't "re-educate" the stomach. If you are trying to lose weight, you also need to learn to eat less at each sitting. Bulk-forming laxatives, unfortunately, train the stomach to expect more food at each meal, not less.

Bulk-forming laxatives containing psyllium, methylcellulose, carboxymethyl cellulose, agar, and karaya gum have no place in weight reduction.

The Pharmacist's Prescription for Weight Reduction

Develop a reasonable weight goal for yourself.

Determine your daily caloric intake *before* starting your diet. Then determine where you can limit your caloric intake.

If your health allows, initiate a regular exercise program along with your diet.

Keep a log of everything you put in your mouth.

Don't change your normal eating pattern if you feel stressed, depressed, or elated.

Don't eat to celebrate every victory or to mourn every loss.

Make sure you are really hungry before you eat. In other words, are you eating because you're hungry or just to be eating?

Consider taking a general purpose multivitamin to maintain your nutrition while you diet.

See the Doctor if . . .

- You are trying to lose more than twenty pounds.
- You are more than sixty years old.
- You are more than forty-five years old and do not exercise much.
- You have any chronic condition, including diabetes, heart disease, high blood pressure, or kidney disease.
- You have chest pains, dizziness, or shortness of breath.
- You intend to increase your daily exercise.

Products Recommended for Self-Treatment of Obesity

None

Products Not Recommended for Self-Treatment of Obesity

Anorexin Capsules (D,E,I)

Appedrine Tablets (D,E,I)

Ayd's AM/PM (D,E,I)

Ayd's Extra Strength (D,E,I)

Caffeine Free Extra Strength Dexatrim (D,E)

Caltrim Diet Plan Capsules (A,D,E,I)

Caltrim Reducing Plan Tablets (A,D,E,I)

Coffee, Tea & A New Me
   (D,E)
Control (D,E)
Dex-A-Diet II (D,E,I)
Dex-A-Diet Lite (D,E)
Dexatrim Capsules
   (D,E,I)
Diadax (D,E,)
Dietac (D,E)
Dietac Sustained Release
   (D,E)
Diet-Trim (A,D,E,I)
Extra Strength Dexatrim
   (D,E,I)

Grapefruit Diet Plan
   (A,D,E,I)
Prolamine Capsules
   (D,E,I)
Slim Line Candy (A,I)
Slime Line Gum (A)
Thinz Back-To-Nature
   (D,E,I)
Thinz Before Meals
   (D,E,I)
Thinz Delite (D,E,I)
Thinz Drops (D,E,I)
Thinz-Span (D,E,I)

The products listed in the "Not Recommended" tables are not recommended by me for one or more of the following reasons: (A) One or more ingredients have been reported to be ineffective or only slightly effective for the product's intended purpose; (B) a more effective product is available; (C) the product advertising or description is likely to heighten consumer expectation beyond actual effectiveness; (D) the product has the potential to cause side effects in the average consumer that are more serious than those generally associated with OTC drugs; (E) the product has the potential to cause serious side effects in persons with specific diseases or disorders; (F) another product is available that is capable of producing the same or nearly the same therapeutic effect without the same risk of side effects; (G) persistent use of the product may cause physical dependency that alters an otherwise normal body function; (H) the product's formulation may reduce the effectiveness of one of its ingredients; (I) this is a multiple-ingredient product that may have no therapeutic advantage over simpler or single-ingredient products; (J) one or more of the product's ingredients may be used for only a short period during the total duration of the illness; (K) the product cannot easily be administered at a dosage level within generally recommended boundaries of optimal therapeutic effect; (L) this is a condition-specific product that is appropriate for use only after a health professional has helped the patient establish a diagnosis.

9

Staying Awake or Going to Sleep

Laugh and the world laughs with you;
Snore and you sleep alone.
—Anthony Burgess (1917–   )

A survey conducted by the American Cancer Society showed that 95 percent of adult Americans claimed to have insomnia at some time in their lives. One of the problems in treating insomnia, however, is that the term means different things to different people.

For some, insomnia may be difficulty in falling asleep; for others, it may be difficulty in staying asleep; and for still others, it may mean awakening too early in the morning. All three of these sleep patterns fall into the category of insomnia, but they all require different treatments.

Many people complain of insomnia and demand treatment when there is no evidence of sleep disorder. You only harm yourself if you self-medicate or demand a prescription from your doctor when you don't have a problem.

So how can you tell if you are getting enough sleep? That's easy enough—your own body will tell you.

The best test of the quality and quantity of your sleep is the way you feel during the day. Let your body be your barometer. If you aren't tired during the day, you don't have a problem. And don't let anyone tell you otherwise.

Don't believe the myth that everybody needs a full eight hours of sleep each night. Some people do well with only four hours of sleep, while others may need as much as twelve.

This is not to say that there is no such thing as insomnia. Almost one-half of American adults have occasional trouble sleeping, while one-third have consistent problems.

Basic Facts About Sleep

Sleep Cycles and Stages

What could be simpler than sleep? You go to bed, close your eyes, and your body takes a break for a few hours, right?

Fifty years ago scientists would have agreed with you. We now know that sleep is an active process composed of various stages of function. In fact, sleep researchers have identified sixty-eight different types of insomnia. This would seem to indicate that the sleep process is more complicated than we would ordinarily think.

What happens when the lights go out?

As you drift off to Slumberland, your brain slowly changes its pace of activity. You first pass through Stage One sleep, the lightest phase. As you relax and place yourself in the care of Hypnos and Morpheus, your brain passes through Stage Two sleep and finally goes into Delta sleep, the deepest and most restful of the sleep stages.

You remain in Stage Two and Delta sleep for most of the night. But sleep is not static. Every sixty to ninety minutes the brain cycles through each of the sleep stages and occasionally ventures into rapid-eye-movement, or REM, sleep.

During REM sleep your eyes dart back and forth beneath the eyelids, muscles become temporarily paralyzed, breathing becomes irregular, heart rate and blood pressure increase, and the stomach pumps more acid. Dreams occur primarily during REM sleep. In young adults REM sleep accounts for about 25 percent of total sleep time. This percentage decreases with age.

After an episode of REM sleep, the brain cycles back down through the sleep stages and repeats the process several times a night.

Sleep-Wake Cycles

Sleep is a fragile thing. Disruption of sleep stages is the cause of only some cases of insomnia. Disturbances of the sleep-wake cycle are common causes of other cases.

The sleep-wake cycle is the pattern of alternating sleep and alertness that each of us develops. For instance, a person may routinely awaken at 6:00 A.M. each morning, stay awake all day, and go to sleep at 11:00 P.M. each evening. This is his normal routine, or sleep-wake cycle. He will probably sleep well as long as this cycle remains constant, but there may be trouble if the routine is disrupted.

Shift workers have a constant battle with their sleep-wake cycles. Some authorities have even referred to insomnia in these people as an occupational disease. People who have to change work schedules frequently (nurses are a good example) never have the opportunity to establish a normal sleep pattern. The same is true of international airline flight crews, who constantly cross time zones.

Our bodies are regulated by an internal "clock." A full clock cycle is about twenty-four hours, but that cycle can drift if we let it. We can't expect to sleep well consistently if we keep irregular hours.

Each of us functions better at particular times of the day. We sleep best at certain times and poorly at others. Some of us are early birds, while others are night owls. Trouble starts when a night owl has to function on an early bird schedule. The reverse is probably an even greater problem.

Age as a Factor in Sleep

Your age is the single most important factor in your sleep pattern. Newborn infants are world champion sleepers. For the first few months after birth they sleep about eighteen hours a day. (But every parent can tell you that they are the wrong eighteen hours!)

As we grow older we sleep less each day, and need less sleep. A four-year-old typically needs ten to twelve hours of sleep per night, while a ten-year-old needs only nine to ten hours. During adolescence sleep requirements drop to about eight hours, and requirements continue to taper off until they reach about six hours in the elderly.

But remember, the amount of time spent sleeping is not as important as how you feel the next day. Some people do fine with only four hours of sleep, while others need ten or twelve. And don't let anyone tell you that you *must* have eight hours of sleep a night—or that you're getting older, so you need more sleep. Forcing yourself to sleep more if you don't need to does not improve your health. You are the only one who can judge your sleep needs.

Causes of Insomnia

There seems to be almost as many causes of insomnia as there are insomniacs. Some of them are listed below. It's beyond the scope of this chapter to discuss them all in any detail; that would require another whole book. But I can briefly describe some of the major causes.

Some Common Causes of Insomnia

Anxiety
Change in work shift
Depression
Dieting
Drinking coffee, tea, or other caffeine-containing beverages
Excessive light
Exercise shortly before bedtime
Fear of insomnia
Fever
Heart disease
Jet lag
Noise
Oversleeping the previous day

Pain, including
Angina
Arthritis
Headache
Muscle ache
Toothache
Ulcers
Respiratory disease
Self-fulfilling prophecies
Smoking
Thyroid disease
Uncomfortable bed
Uncomfortable temperature or humidity
Withdrawal from alcohol or sleeping pills

Pain

One of the two most common causes of sleeplessness is pain. We cannot relax when we are in pain, and the ability to relax is critical to good sleep. The origin of the pain doesn't matter, but the intensity does.

If you have difficulty sleeping because of pain, don't reach for a sleeping pill. Some studies performed several years ago indicated that sleeping medications can actually *increase* pain perceptions. You would be better off to treat the cause of the pain rather than to medicate the sleeplessness.

Emotional Difficulties

The other leading cause of insomnia is emotional stress, anxiety. People who take their worries to bed have a difficult time getting to sleep. And the sleep they do get is of very poor quality.

Depression, anxiety's first cousin, also disrupts sleep, but in a different way. People with severe depression may have difficulty getting to sleep, but more commonly they experience a condition called "early morning waking." These folks sleep poorly through the night and then wake up two or three hours before their normal waking time. They may be unable to get back to sleep and usually feel terrible for the rest of the day. The pattern of poor sleep and daytime fatigue contributes to their feelings of depression and disrupts their sleep again the next night.

Self-administration of sleeping pills isn't the answer for these people either. They need a good therapist and a doctor's supervision for their sleep problems.

Irregular Schedules

I have already mentioned shift work and jet lag as causes of sleep-wake cycle problems. But have you ever considered oversleeping as a cause of insomnia?

Those who have this problem are "sleep gourmets." They relish the exquisite pleasure of sleep and delay arising until they consume the last succulent morsel of rest.

People who make a habit of "sleeping out" each day are headed for trouble when they try to go to sleep the next night. Their problem is that they can only sleep so many hours each day. By lingering in bed they reset their internal clock, which causes the body to delay sleep onset at night. This delay makes them feel even more tired the next morning, and the problem perpetuates itself.

Hormone Imbalances

Hormone imbalances may also disturb sleep. Excess secretion of the adrenal glands as well as too much or too little thyroid hormone disturb sleep patterns. Once again, the treatment of these conditions rests with your doctor, not with self-medication.

Sleeping Environment

Just as pain can cause you to lose sleep, any other body discomfort can disrupt your rest. Sleeping in an uncomfortable bed provides a constant annoyance, as does too much noise or light in the bedroom.

Taken as a group, people have wide tolerances to nighttime noises. While some need absolute quiet to get to sleep, others like to be lulled to sleep by music or voices on radio or television. Women seem to be more sensitive to noises than men. A mother can hear a baby cry in the next county, while some dads can sleep right through a tornado.

One of the most misunderstood environmental factors is room temperature. It's difficult to sleep in a hot room. Most people know that they sleep poorly when room temperature rises about 75 degrees, but they don't know that the same happens when the temperature is uncomfortably cool.

So-called "good sleeping weather" is usually bad sleeping weather. It feels good to snuggle under the blankets if you awaken during the night when the air is nippy. If this feels so good, how can it be bad weather to sleep in?

The problem is that the cool temperatures awaken you from your normal sleep. You have to wake up before you can "feel good." This waking fragments your sleep, messes up your sleep stages, and deprives you of your normal amount of sleep during the night. But, again, the real test is how you feel the next day.

If you pay attention the next time you have "good sleeping weather," you'll probably notice that you were pretty tired the next day. This doesn't sound so good after all, does it?

Try to change your sleeping environment if it is causing you to sleep poorly. Eliminate or reduce light and noise when possible. Control the temperature to between 65 degrees and 75 degrees as best you can. Humidity that is uncomfortably high or low can also affect your breathing and disturb your sleep.

Try to maintain a comfortable environment in the bedroom.

Hunger

Hunger is another comfort-related problem. Dieters who go to bed hungry have difficulty getting to sleep because the quiet of the bedroom allows them to focus all their attention on their empty stomachs. At the other extreme, overeaters can experience indigestion when they lie down. (This effect is described in chapter 5.)

If you are dieting, you might try to save some of your caloric allotment for a bedtime snack. But don't eat a big meal or spicy foods before retiring, because lying down may force your stomach to regurgitate food into the esophagus.

Illness

Illnesses can disturb sleep patterns. Infections and fever may increase sleep time but decrease sleep quality. Heart and blood vessel diseases such as angina, congestive heart failure, and hardening of the arteries all decrease sleep. Respiratory disorders like asthma attacks, emphysema, and chronic bronchitis also disrupt sleep because of the constant battle to keep breathing.

Fear of Insomnia

The *fear* of insomnia may itself cause insomnia. People who have this fear are terrified by the thought that they may not be able to sleep. Often they predict that they can't sleep if they spend the night away from home. Or they may fear that change in daily routine is affecting their sleep. Some also insist that they can't sleep if they don't take sleeping pills.

All of these fears turn into self-fulfilling prophecies. Those who fear insomnia first *predict* that they will not sleep, and then they become upset over the *prospect* of not sleeping. Their anxieties prevent them from sleeping, thus fulfilling their predictions. These people usually need counseling rather than medication.

Medications

Use of medication can also cause sleep disturbances. It should be obvious that stimulant drugs can disrupt sleep. After all, we take them to stay awake or improve our function during the day. Caffeine is the most commonly used stimulant, but other drugs have stimulant properties of which you may not be aware. Theophylline and aminophylline, used for asthma and other respiratory problems, have stimulant side effects. So do the decongestants that you may take for a cold.

If you have difficulty sleeping at night, it would be a good idea for you to consult your pharmacist before starting to take any new drug. You might also want him or her to review the other medications that you have been taking all along.

Ironically, the drugs that most predictably cause sleep problems are sleeping pills themselves! Prescription sleeping pills, technically called hypnotics, are proven to disrupt sleep stages and diminish REM sleep. Most of them have also been shown to lose their effect with continuous use, some in as little as three days!

They may also cause hangover effects the next morning.

As if that weren't bad enough, most, if not all, of these drugs are addicting.

One of the reasons people think they need sleep medications forever is that they experience *rebound insomnia* when they try to stop taking them. This rebound effect is frequently an early symptom of a drug withdrawal reaction. I've known people who continued to take these medications for years, not because the drugs still worked, but because these people would go through drug withdrawal if they stopped taking them!

If that's the case, how did these drugs get to be so popular? I think it's probably because we health professionals did not recognize the drugs' limitations until recent years. However, that's no excuse for starting new patients on these drugs now. There is more than enough evidence in the medical literature to warn pharmacists and physicians about their disadvantages. Very few people are candidates for sleeping medications. However, prescribing a "sleeper" for a patient is usually easier than determining the cause of insomnia and recommending methods to combat it.

If you have *consistent* difficulty sleeping, do not hesitate to see your doctor. However, if he or she simply suggests medication, ask for a referral to a sleep disorders center. There are forty-one such centers accredited by the Association of Sleep Disorders Centers, and your doctor should be able to refer you to one.

Don't let friends or television advertisers convince you to take medication you don't need. Most people need only five minutes to settle down and fall asleep, but others, especially those over sixty years old, may routinely need fifteen to twenty minutes. There is nothing wrong with waiting twenty minutes to get to sleep. Don't medicate problems that don't exist!

Nicotine and Alcohol

Unfortunately, stimulants and hypnotics aren't the only drugs that disturb sleep. Nicotine and alcohol can do a number on you, too. The nicotine in tobacco is a stimulant drug that we tend to overlook. Heavy cigarette smokers don't sleep as well as nonsmokers. Improved sleep is one of the hidden or undercover benefits of kicking the habit.

Alcohol has both beneficial and detrimental effects on sleep. A drink before bedtime can help you relax, but several drinks may put you under before you get under the sheets.

Alcohol is a double-edged sword, a poor choice as a nighttime sedative. Like sleeping pills, it disrupts your sleep stages and the sleep you get is not restful. In addition, alcohol can wake you up and cause uncomfortable tremors when your body begins to clear the alcohol from your system. Overall, you may sleep less with alcohol than if you waited to get to sleep naturally.

Resolving Sleep Difficulties

Improving Sleep Without Drugs

Drugs certainly may be used to help you get to sleep, but you may end up with more problems than you started with. It has been my experience that the great majority of people who have difficulty sleeping can improve their situation simply by analyzing their problems and either doing something about those problems themselves or seeking expert help.

The first step in improving your sleep is to determine the reason for your sleeplessness. For instance, if you are in the habit of drinking a cup of coffee shortly before bedtime, try substituting decaffeinated coffee or a soft drink that does not contain caffeine.

That's pretty obvious, but some problems are not so simple.

Many people with sleep problems don't get sufficient exercise during the day to make them tired at night. The answer to this is to increase your exercise, right?

Well, maybe. Exercise is a funny thing. It can either improve or wreck your sleep. If you don't get enough exercise during the day, you don't burn off the body's energy stores and you aren't tired at bedtime. If you try to exercise right before bedtime, you key up your body for action just when you want to go to sleep. *Exercising just before bedtime can stimulate your body and your mind for as long as two hours.*

The trick is to engage in some physical activity during the day—but long enough before bedtime to prevent it from disturbing your sleep. As a general rule, I advise patients to complete their exercise routines at least four hours before they intend to go to bed.

The afternoon nap is a deadly practice for those with sleep problems. Your body will allow you to sleep only so many hours per twenty-four-hour period. *If you want to sleep better at night, don't sleep during the day.*

This is especially troublesome for the elderly. Friends, relatives, and television sitcoms tell them that they should sleep all day. When they try cat-napping through the day, they often find that they cannot sleep at night. What good does that do?

Sleep only when you are tired and only for as long as necessary. If you tire during the day, take a nap. But don't expect to sleep as much at night as you otherwise would.

Regular routine is essential for those of you who have problems with your sleep-wake cycles. If you have a bad night, make sure you still get up at your regular time. This will help you do better the next night. Also, try to establish a regular bedtime.

The combination of a regular bedtime with a regular waking time can do wonders. It may seem like torture at first, but you should see benefits after a few days.

Some people live in the bedroom. They eat meals there, they watch television there, they do their exercises on the bedroom floor, they knit or read in bed. And then they wonder why they can't sleep.

Your mind needs exercise as much as your body. If you stay cooped up all day in your bedroom, your brain can't tell when it's time for sleep. You should only do two things in the bedroom. And one of them is sleep.

Your psychological preparation for sleep is also important. If you have persistent problems with insomnia, you might take a tip from the pediatricians. They tell us that the best way to get children ready for bed is to institute "quiet time" about an hour before bedtime. Quiet time is a period when we read books to the kids or tell stories. The whole idea is to relax both the body and mind, thus allowing the child to wind down before going to bed. The same principle works for adults.

Try to relax and prepare yourself for bed. Quiet time is enjoyable even if you don't have sleep problems. The activities you choose are up to you, but reading and listening to music are two of my favorites. You might want to work on your hobby, take a warm bath, write letters, or engage in some other relaxing activity. You may do whatever you like, but I don't recommend paying the monthly bills or talking to your mother-in-law.

All of the preceding advice is fine if you are trying to prevent a sleepless night, but what do you do if you go to bed and *then* discover that you can't sleep? It's a little late for exercise or abstaining from caffeine, isn't it?

True, but there are still some things you can do.

One of the worst things you can do to yourself is to lie in bed and stare at the ceiling. Pretty soon you'll start to get frustrated and angry with yourself for not going to sleep. If you feel this happening, get up out of bed and go to another room. Once you're out of bed you can try the quiet time routine. Listen to some soft music or read a magazine or book. Usually, boring reading material is better than more interesting stuff. When I was a student, pharmaceutical chemistry textbooks did the job for me.

Some people find that warm milk works for them. Personally, I find the taste of warm milk revolting. The interesting thing about warm milk is that it works, but not for the reason you might expect.

Warm milk has no magical properties. Sleep scientists find that it is no more effective in inducing sleep than a placebo. What works is the process, rather than the milk. When we are frustrated at our inability to sleep, we get up, putter around the kitchen a bit, get out the milk and a saucepan, and slowly heat and stir the milk until it is sufficiently warm. We pour the milk into a glass or cup, sit in a comfortable chair, and slowly sip.

That sounds like quiet time to me.

Nonprescription Sleep Aids

If your sleep problem has not improved after following the measures just described, there is little chance that the OTC drugs will help you, either.

Antihistamines—Drugs That Deliver Sleep as an Occasional Side Effect

Most OTC products for sleep difficulties simply contain an antihistamine. Since drowsiness is a common side effect of antihistamines, they may help to put you to sleep. However, since sedation is only a side effect, not a primary effect of the antihistamines, you may suspect that this effect will probably not be very pronounced or last very long. In either case you would be correct.

We know that not everyone experiences drowsiness after taking a dose of antihistamine. We also know that people develop resistance to antihistamine-induced drowsiness after a few doses.

That doesn't make these products sound too good, does it?

That's why I don't recommend any of them.

Purchasing these sleep aids not only separates you from your money, but the drugs themselves are potentially hazardous. All of the warnings about possible antihistamine side effects given in chapter 2 apply to the use of these drugs. In addition, people who do not fall asleep after one dose of an OTC nighttime sedative may be tempted to pop a few more doses. After all, these are only OTC drugs and are safe, right?

No. They're only safe if used properly. Antihistamine overdoses are dangerous. Overdoses can cause headache, nausea, irregular heartbeat, nervousness, hallucinations, fever, and seizures. If you insist on using these things, take them correctly. Read all label directions carefully; don't exceed recommended doses. And keep these drugs away from the kids. An antihistamine overdose in a child can be deadly.

Tryptophan—An Unproven Fad Medication

Tryptophan is one of the current darlings of the health food industry. It doesn't seem to matter that this amino acid has not been proven to be effective for treating insomnia.

The legend of tryptophan began curiously enough with the warm-milk-at-bedtime myth. Since warm milk (I still don't understand why it has to be *warm)* was supposed to be so effective for inducing sleep, chemists made a search for the sleep-producing chemical. The search ended with the discovery of the amino acid tryptophan. Scientists already knew that tryptophan was a chemical precursor to serotonin, a chemical in the brain that is thought to produce sleep. So they thought they had a safe and natural sleep-producing substance.

As it turns out, while tryptophan is required to form serotonin in the brain, so are a lot of other things. And serotonin isn't the only chemical that is required for sleep.

Unfortunately, the whole tryptophan thing has gotten out of hand. Tryptophan is not approved by the FDA for use in sleep disorders. Why not? Because no one has definitely proven that the stuff works. Therefore, tryptophan can only be legally sold as a dietary supplement, not as a sleep aid. And I doubt that this status will ever change.

The Pharmacist's Prescription for Insomnia

Most cases of insomnia are annoying but not disabling. Don't complicate sleeplessness by self-medicating.

Try to determine the cause of your insomnia and take steps to prevent further episodes.

If you cannot sleep, get up and try some of the "quiet time" techniques mentioned earlier in this chapter.

Avoid caffeine-containing beverages in the evening.

Don't eat a large meal just before bedtime, but don't go to bed hungry either. Try eating a light snack if you are hungry.

Establish your own personal "quiet time" routine.

Get up at about the same time each day.
Go to bed at about the same time every night.
Keep work- or stress-related material out of the bedroom.
Increase your daytime physical activity.
Listen to relaxing music.
Read a boring book or magazine before bedtime.
Reduce noise and light in the bedroom.
Take a warm bath before going to bed.

See the Doctor if . . .

- You have loss of sleep plus lack of energy, weight loss, weight gain, anxiety, or decreased sex drive.
- You feel depressed and continually wake up too early in the morning.
- Your sleep has not improved in two weeks despite using drug or nondrug therapies.
- Your sleep problem is due to a medical problem, such as pain, heart disease, or breathing difficulties.

Products Recommended for Self-Treatment of Insomnia
None

Daytime Sedative or Stimulant Needs

Daytime Tension

Stress, anxiety, and "simple nervous tension" are all close relatives of insomnia. In many cases they are simply different manifestations of the same disorder. We used to see commercials for products intended to treat these problems, but they don't seem to be aired anymore. Why not? Because the FDA found that these products were neither safe nor effective for treatment of stress. On June 22, 1979, all of them were ordered off the market.

If that's the case why are Compoz, Nervine, and the others still on store shelves?

By this time you should be aware that OTC drug products have more lives than a cat. The manufacturers of these products simply changed the ingredients and relabeled them for use as *nighttime sedatives!*

For the record, there are no FDA-approved daytime sedatives on the OTC market. Nor will there be any in the foreseeable future.

If you are troubled with undue anxiety or tension, your best bet is to see a counselor.

Daytime Fatigue

Daytime fatigue is a common problem. Those who have insomnia frequently need something to get them going the next day. In addition, people with boring or tedious jobs may also need help to keep them alert and attentive.

People with medical disorders such as heart failure, infections, anemia, hormone problems, and muscle diseases may feel drained and tired much of the day. In other cases, medications may cause drowsiness and interfere with daytime activity.

For years the pharmaceutical industry has been searching for safe and effective stimulants, but their track record hasn't been too good. The closest they came was with the development of amphetamine but that caused more problems than it was worth.

Caffeine—The Best Available Stimulant

There is no perfect stimulant on the market, either as a prescription or nonprescription drug. The best alternative right now is caffeine.

Caffeine is the only stimulant that meets the FDA advisory panel's requirements for safety and efficacy. Doses should not exceed 200 milligrams every three hours, and doses that high should not be taken for more than two weeks at a time.

The good news about caffeine is that you don't have to buy a drug product to get it. The bad news is that you can experience some very uncomfortable side effects if you take a caffeine-containing drug in addition to your regular coffee or tea intake.

Americans consume over 15 million pounds of caffeine per year, most of it in beverages. For instance, a cup of brewed coffee contains 100 to 150 milligrams of caffeine, twelve ounces of cola contain 40 to 70 milligrams, a cup of tea contains 60 to 70 milligrams, and a cup of cocoa has about 50 milligrams.

Compare those "doses" with a Nodoz tablet that contains 100 milligrams of caffeine and you will see that two cups of your morning coffee can easily give you more caffeine than the recommended dose of Nodoz. There is no need to take OTC stimulants if you enjoy drinking coffee or tea during the day.

Caffeine is a stimulant that occurs in nature, but that doesn't make it free of side effects. Doses over 250 milligrams (two cups of brewed coffee) can stimulate the heart muscle and cause irregular heartbeat in people with heart disease. People who drink six cups of coffee per day double their chances of heart attack in comparison to those who don't drink coffee at all.

Caffeine also affects the nervous system. In small amounts it stimulates thought processes and improves muscle coordination, but in amounts larger than 250 milligrams it can cause restlessness, tremors, and headache. And *never drink coffee at bedtime*. It can cause insomnia.

The kidneys aren't spared, either. Caffeine is a mild diuretic—that is, it increases urine production. This is an effect that is well known to every coffee drinker.

But how good a stimulant is it? Unfortunately, you don't get something for nothing. The stimulation that caffeine gives you draws on your body's energy reserves. When the effects of the caffeine wear off, you frequently are in worse shape than you were before.

Recommended Stimulants

Amostat tablets	Quick-Pep tablets
Caffedrine capsules	Tirend tablets
Nodoz tablets	Wakoz

All of the above contain 200 milligrams or less of caffeine as the active ingredient. They should not be taken in addition to caffeine-containing beverages.

Stimulants Not Recommended for Self-Medication

Pep-Back (I)   Vivarin (I)
Summit (I)

Or the generic equivalent of any of the above

The products listed in the "Not Recommended" tables are not recommended by me for one or more of the following reasons: (A) One or more ingredients have been reported to be ineffective or only slightly effective for the product's intended purpose; (B) a more effective product is available; (C) the product advertising or description is likely to heighten consumer expectation beyond actual effectiveness; (D) the product has the potential to cause side effects in the average consumer that are more serious than those generally associated with OTC drugs; (E) the product has the potential to cause serious side effects in persons with specific diseases or disorders; (F) another product is available that is capable of producing the same or nearly the same therapeutic effect without the same risk of side effects; (G) persistent use of the product may cause physical dependency that alters an otherwise normal body function; (H) the product's formulation may reduce the effectiveness of one of its ingredients; (I) this is a multiple-ingredient product that may have no therapeutic advantage over simpler or single-ingredient products; (J) one or more of the product's ingredients may be used for only a short period during the total duration of the illness; (K) the product cannot easily be administered at a dosage level within generally recommended boundaries of optimal therapeutic effect; (L) this is a condition-specific product that is appropriate for use only after a health professional has helped the patient establish a diagnosis.

10

What Can You Believe About Vitamins and Minerals?

> The only way to keep your health
> is to eat what you don't want,
> drink what you don't like
> and do what you'd rather not.
> —Mark Twain (1835–1910)

True or false?

- Vitamins prevent hair loss.
- Vitamins help you sleep better.
- Vitamins improve your sex drive.
- Vitamins prevent infections.
- Vitamins improve your skin.
- Vitamins prevent stress.
- Vitamins improve your appetite.
- Vitamins prevent mosquito bites.

Sad though it may be, all of these claims are false. But I'm sure you know people who seem to have experienced some of these effects. Placebos, inert "medications," can also produce all of these effects. This is what makes the use, misuse, and profiteering from vitamins so confusing.

Caveat Emptor—Buyer Beware!

There is nothing wrong with marketing and profit-making, unless they are accomplished under false pretenses or with misinformation. That often is the case with vitamins.

Americans consume vitamins and nutritional supplements way out of proportion to these products' true value. People fall victim to claims that organic vitamins are the only ones to use (*all* vitamins are organic), that natural vitamins are superior to synthetic (your body can't tell the difference), and that you can't overdose on vitamins because they're natural (you can overdose on water, and that's natural, too).

The "stress formula" vitamins are one example of how vitamin advertisers mislead you. Stress, advertisers claim, has been proven to increase your body's need for vitamins. That's true, as far as the statement goes. However, the researchers who discovered the link between stress and vitamins were not talking about *emotional* stress; they were referring to *physical* stresses, such as fever, infections, broken bones, and other physical maladies.

Likewise, the term *natural* is often linked with vitamins, usually to consumers' detriment. *Natural* is supposed to mean that the vitamin comes from a plant or animal source rather than a chemical laboratory.

Your body cannot tell the difference between an expensive "natural" vitamin and an economical synthetic one. Sometimes vitamin products touted as "natural" are supplemented with synthetic vitamins! Or a vitamin may be chemically extracted from its plant source, concentrated into a chemically pure form, and then incorporated into a vitamin tablet, all the while being called "natural."

More upsetting to me than the misleading information on vitamin sources are the extreme claims made for vitamin effects. People gulp handfuls of vitamin tablets and capsules and guzzle tonics in the belief that vitamin B_{12} will give them extra energy, vitamin C will protect them from colds, or vitamin E will improve their sex life.

None of this is true.

The Legal Status of Claims for Supplements— Where Is the FDA?

People think they are better protected by federal regulations than they really are. Federal legislation, in particular the Proxmire Amendment, requires that any regulation of the potency of vitamin and mineral products be based on considerations of toxicity rather than physical need. In other words, the FDA cannot stop the sale of vitamins or minerals that are worthless unless they can also prove that they are harmful. Nor can they halt the sale of high-dose vitamins unless these same products can be shown to cause undue toxicity. While the FDA can still protect us to some degree from dangerous doses of vitamins, it cannot protect us from false claims.

That doesn't sound like consumer protection to me.

The FDA also labors under another serious restriction. If a manufacturer of a vitamin or mineral product does not make medical claims on the label of the product, the FDA has to consider it as a food rather than a drug. (The FDA's food standards are much less stringent than those it applies to drugs.) In other words, a manufacturer can state on his label that his brand of vitamin C is effective for treatment or prevention of vitamin C deficiency, but if he states that it prevents colds, the FDA can pull his product off the market.

Consequently, today's vitamin hucksters have to be discreet about advertising practices. Since they can't advertise unproven claims directly, they have to find other means to spread the word. And they seem to do this effectively through consumer-oriented magazines and word-of-mouth advertising.

This is not to say that all false vitamin claims are intentionally misleading. Many are well-intentioned but misinformed.

Who Can You Trust to Tell the Truth About Vitamins?

Vitamin ''experts'' are generally polarized into two factions. One group seems to believe that the benefits of vitamins and minerals are endless and that the more you take the better you'll feel. On the other side are the conservatives, who question every claim for vitamin efficacy, even those that have been tentatively proven.

The truth about vitamins is probably somewhere in the middle ground.

I believe that much of the popularity of vitamins is due to the desire to treat oneself rather than hand one's medical care over completely to someone else. Vitamins offer us a way to do this. After all, vitamins are natural, and natural substances can't hurt us, right?

Wrong. Anything, natural or otherwise, taken in excess can be harmful. Too much sunshine, exercise, or alcohol (yes, alcohol is a natural product, too) can be harmful, even fatal.

Where can you go for reliable information on vitamins and nutrition? It would seem that a nutritionist would be a good source, but that isn't always the case. The problem with choosing nutritionists is that they don't have to have any special education or background at all! *You* could be a nutritionist if you wanted. Just hang out a shingle and suddenly you're a nutritionist, too!

To be perfectly candid, most health professionals don't have extensive training in nutrition, either. Fortunately, there is one group that does—registered dietitians.

At a minimum, dietitians must have a Bachelor of Science degree in foods and nutrition, plus a period of internship. Many dietitians also have Master's degrees and supervised work experience.

But that in itself does not qualify dietitians to do nutritional counseling. In order to be "registered" they must pass an examination prepared and administered by the American Dietetic Association (ADA) in Chicago. And the process does not even end there. In order to maintain their registration, registered dietitians also have to participate regularly in continuing education programs and report their continuing education credits to the ADA.

"Nutritionists" are not subject to such quality controls.

What You Don't Know About Supplements *Can* Hurt You

Uncritical and indiscriminate use of vitamins and nutritional supplements can do more than lighten your wallet; it can also damage your health.

The idea that natural remedies can prevent illness or restore health and vitality is attractive, but it seldom works that way. Overuse of vitamins may cause side effects or toxic reactions. People who use vitamins for self-treatment of self-diagnosed disorders often delay proper diagnosis of treatable conditions.

Misconceptions about the role of vitamins in health

abound. One survey showed that 75 percent of those interviewed believed that vitamin supplements can supply energy. This is a basic misconception. It is *impossible* for vitamins to directly provide energy to a person who is not vitamin deficient. Another study indicated that 20 percent of people believe that cancer and arthritis are caused by vitamin and mineral deficits. These surveys illustrate how poorly some people understand the role of vitamins in nutrition.

Vitamins are only facilitators. They are necessary in small amounts for the normal metabolic functions of the body. With few exceptions, amounts in excess of your body's basic needs contribute no additional benefit.

Vitamins are like the oil in your car. If you have no oil, the car will not run at all. If you have some but not enough oil, the car will run for a while but develop problems. If you have the proper amount of oil, the car will run well, but if you overload the system with oil, the engine will choke and gag until it gets rid of the excess.

Many people believe that vitamins are harmless because they are natural. Not so. Natural substances can be just as toxic as synthetic ones. After all, strychnine and cyanide are natural. And when you were a Girl or Boy Scout weren't you warned not to eat any wild berries or mushrooms you couldn't identify?

Being "natural" is no guarantee of safety. Neither is it an assurance that a synthetic drug won't work better.

In writing this chapter I have applied the same standards to vitamins and minerals that I have to the drugs discussed in each of the other chapters. This may not be popular among the vitamin fanatics, who don't consider vitamins to be drugs even though they use them as drugs.

There has to be some degree of uniformity in assessing and judging the value of *all* therapeutic agents, or we never will be able to separate the drugs and vitamins that work from those that don't. If we ignore uniformity and objectivity, we become easy prey for the charlatans and quacks.

What Is a Vitamin?

One of the sources of confusion over nutrition is that people don't seem to understand what distinguishes the various nutrients. While most people feel that they know what a vitamin is, many, in fact, do not. This confusion is the reason that some vitamin proponents get away with claiming that laetrile and other worthless and potentially dangerous compounds are "vitamins."

Simply stated, a vitamin is an organic chemical substance required in small amounts for the normal metabolic function of the body but not produced in the body in sufficient quantities to carry out this function.

A chemical doesn't become a vitamin just because some self-proclaimed nutritionist says so. A chemical is not a vitamin until it is proven to be essential for normal function.

Understanding RDA

Some vitamin enthusiasts promote "megadoses" of vitamins for various purposes. A megadose is a dose at least ten times larger than the RDA for that vitamin.

So what's an RDA? RDA is an abbreviation for "Recommended Dietary Allowance," an estimate of the *total* quantities of vitamins a normal, healthy person should ingest from all sources (both from diet and vitamin supplements) in an average day. The RDA's are determined by the Committee on Dietary Allowances of the Food and Nutrition Board. They are designed so that the levels recommended are thought to be above actual needs for 80 percent of people but are still safe for 100 percent of the healthy population.

The Food and Nutrition Board is responsible for revising and publishing updated RDA's every five years. Unfortunately, as this is written in 1986, the Committee on Dietary Allowances still has not been able to agree on the 1985 revision and the 1980 RDA's are still in effect. The RDA's listed for vitamins in this chapter are, therefore, 1980 RDA's.

A simplified version of the RDA is the U.S.R.D.A., or United States Recommended Daily Allowance. These are the percentage values you find on the labels of vitamin products. They can be used as a guide for comparing one vitamin product with another.

Who Needs Vitamins?

The notion that everyone needs vitamin supplements is not true. If you have an adequate diet, you don't need additional vitamins. The problem lies in determining whether you are eating an adequate diet.

If you normally eat an average of 2500 to 3000 calories per day and balance your diet among the four major food groups—dairy products, meat and fish, vegetables and fruits, and bread and cereals—you probably don't need to take the vitamin tablets. However, if your diet dips below 2000 calories per day, it becomes difficult to maintain an adequate vitamin intake.

One survey indicates that the average woman between the ages of thirty-five and forty-four consumes only 1440 calories daily. A woman eating this way probably needs a multivitamin supplement.

Others who may need extra vitamins include heavy alcohol drinkers, those on special diets (especially vegetarian or weight reduction diets), pregnant women and nursing mothers, people with intestinal diseases that impair food digestion and nutrient absorption, and those who take prescription medications that interfere with vitamins in the body.

Are Vitamins Nutrients or Drugs?

That depends on how much you take.

Vitamins are essential to life. You cannot survive long without them. In this context, vitamins are nutrients and have few side effects. However, vitamins taken in excessive quantities are an entirely different matter.

Some of the vitamin freaks would have us believe that vitamins can be taken in megadoses without risk of toxicity. Their reasoning is that vitamins are our friends, and that therefore they are incapable of doing harm.

Nonsense!

Megadoses of vitamins are drugs, not nutrients. When you take quantities of vitamins far in excess of your body's needs, you are using those vitamins as drugs. And all drugs have side effects.

Nor is there convincing evidence that excess consumption of any one or any combination of nutrients provides extra health benefits to the average person. However, the claims for efficacy of megadoses are attractive to those who seek to prevent or treat incurable or untreatable diseases.

The claims for megavitamins are either unsubstantiated or outright disproven. Two examples of these include the use of niacin for schizophrenia and vitamin C for the common cold. Despite years of investigation, these claims have been impossible to substantiate.

A few genetically based diseases do respond to high doses of vitamins. But before you take such massive doses you need a doctor's diagnosis to determine if you have one of these rare disorders.

Is everyone who promotes high dose vitamins evil? No, usually just misinformed. The problem is that most people don't understand how the body works and how people are different from each other.

When you took high school chemistry, you learned that you always got the same reaction when you mixed the same two chemicals in a test tube, as long as all the variables of concentration, temperature, pressure, and so forth stayed constant. But if you varied one of the conditions of the experiment, you might or might not get the same reaction.

The body is similar to a test tube, but instead of the few variables that you deal with in the laboratory, there are thousands of variables in the body. So on the basis of only one or a few tests, you cannot assume that a drug or vitamin is effective for your intended purpose.

Before a pharmaceutical manufacturer can introduce a new prescription drug onto the market, or even get the FDA to approve a new use for an old drug, the company must show the results of its tests. Usually the testing involves giving the drug to thousands of laboratory animals and human volunteers and carefully noting their response. On the average, the process takes seven years to complete.

The test product is approved for marketing only after it has been shown to perform consistently better than a placebo, or inert, control. Do the megavitamin proponents subject their ideas and theories to such rigid testing? No, they don't. When others try to apply these standards, the megavitamins don't measure up.

Vitamins That Aren't

Since there is so much confusion over what a vitamin is and what it is not, it's relatively easy to "discover" a new vitamin and promote its use for some ill-defined purpose. Some of these phony vitamins are necessary for health but don't fit the definition of a vitamin. Some of them have no nutritional value at all. Still others are outright dangerous. Some of these are listed below. For example, chemical analysis of four brands of pangamic acid, so-called vitamin B_{15}, showed that two brands contained known cancer-producing chemicals. This is what we are forced to put up with since Congress tied the FDA's hands in dealing with vitamins and their manufacturers and promoters.

Non-Vitamins

Aminopurine (vitamin B_4)
Amygdalin (vitamin B_{17}, laetrile)
Arachidonic acid
Bifidus factor
Biopterin
Carnitine
Cholesterol
Chlorophyll
Dimethyl sulfonium (vitamin U)
Hematin
Inositol
Lecithin

Linolenic acid (vitamin F)
Nerve growth factor
Orotic acid (vitamin B_{13})
Pangamic acid (vitamin B_{15})
Para-aminobenzoic acid (vitamin H, PABA)
Pimelic acid
Pteridines
Taurine
Thioctic acid
Ubiquinone (coenzyme Q)
Xanthopterin (vitamin B_{14})

Water-Soluble Vitamins

The B vitamins and vitamin C comprise the water-soluble vitamins. The B vitamins, also known as B complex, are a heterogeneous group. They tend to be found in the same types of foods, and the symptoms of deficiency of the various B complex vitamins are similar. Deficiency of one of these vitamins seldom occurs alone; a person who is deficient in one of them is usually deficient in others.

Since this is only a chapter on vitamins, not a vitamin book, we'll look primarily at some of the more popular OTC vitamins.

Vitamin B$_1$

Thiamine, or vitamin B$_1$, is essential for carbohydrate metabolism, and the amount of thiamine needed increases if dietary carbohydrate increases.

Alcoholism accounts for more causes of thiamine deficiency in the United States than does any other cause. Many alcoholics neglect their diet in pursuit of alcohol and other drugs. As a consequence, they are at risk of developing the complications of thiamine deficiency listed in the table. The most serious of these for an alcoholic is the Wernicke-Korsakoff syndrome. This disorder is characterized by nerve damage that may present itself as psychosis or loss of contact with reality. The nerve damage may be permanent if treatment is not started soon enough. Some of these patients have to be institutionalized for the rest of their lives.

One of the more unusual supposed uses of thiamine is as a mosquito repellant. Some claim that a dose of 100 milligrams of thiamine taken three times a day for three or more days prior to an outing in the woods will prevent mosquito bites. Unfortunately, controlled studies have not been able to prove that this actually happens. There is no harm in trying thiamine for this purpose, as long as you continue to use your usual insect repellant. If you try to rely on thiamine alone, you could end up with more bites than you otherwise would have.

Vitamin B₁

Other Names:
Aneurine hydrochloride
Thiamin hydrochloride
Thiamine chloride
Thiamine hydrochloride
Thiaminium chloride hydrochloride

Proven functions:
Essential for proper nerve function
Necessary for carbohydrate metabolism

Recommended Dietary Allowance (1980):

Infants up to 6 months	0.3 mg.
Infants 6 months to 1 year	0.5 mg.
Children 1 to 3 years	0.7 mg.
Children 4 to 6 years	0.9 mg.
Children 7 to 10 years	1.2 mg.
Males 11 to 14 years	1.4 mg.
Males 15 to 18 years	1.4 mg.
Males 19 to 22 years	1.5 mg.
Males 23 to 50 years	1.4 mg.
Males 51 years and over	1.2 mg.
Females 11 to 14 years	1.1 mg.
Females 15 to 18 years	1.1 mg.
Females 19 to 22 years	1.1 mg.
Females 23 to 50 years	1.0 mg.
Females 51 years and over	1.0 mg.
Pregnant women	*add* 0.4 mg.
Breast-feeding women	*add* 0.5 mg.

Greater amounts of vitamin may be needed in:
• Heavy alcohol consumption
• Heavy carbohydrate consumption
• Use of a kidney machine

Symptoms of deficiency:
Confusion   Difficulty breathing
Diarrhea or
   constipation

Enlarged heart
Fatigue
Heart failure
Irritability
Increased blood
  pressure
Loss of appetite
Loss of manual
  dexterity

Psychosis
Tingling or numbness
  in the hands or feet
Water retention

Some dietary sources:

Bacon
Beans
Cheese
Fortified bread or flour
Fortified breakfast
  cereal
Leafy vegetables

Peas
Wheat germ
Whole-wheat bread or
  flour
Yeast

Unproven uses:

Treatment or prevention of

Anxiety
Cancer
Depression
Diarrhea
Drug side effects

Infections
Mosquito bites
Multiple sclerosis
Senility
Skin rashes

Side effects:

Usually nontoxic, even in high doses
Serious side effects have occurred when thiamine was
  given by injection.

Vitamin B₂

Riboflavin, vitamin B_2, plays an important role in cellular respiration and hydrogen and oxygen utilization. It is also necessary for fatty acid metabolism.

Riboflavin deficiency rarely occurs alone. Therefore, riboflavin is rarely needed as a single vitamin supplement. Riboflavin deficiencies are usually treated with B complex combination products.

Vitamin B₂

Other names:
    Lactoflavin
    Riboflavin
    Vitamin G

Proven functions:
    Essential for growth of cells
    Necessary for utilization of hydrogen, oxygen, and fatty acids in cells
    Constituent of liver enzymes responsible for drug metabolism

Recommended Dietary Allowance (1980):

Infants up to 6 months	0.4 mg.
Infants 6 months to 1 year	0.6 mg.
Children 1 to 3 years	0.8 mg.
Children 4 to 6 years	1.0 mg.
Children 7 to 10 years	1.4 mg.
Males 11 to 14 years	1.6 mg.
Males 15 to 18 years	1.7 mg.
Males 19 to 22 years	1.7 mg.
Males 23 to 50 years	1.6 mg.
Males 51 years and over	1.4 mg.
Females 11 to 14 years	1.3 mg.
Females 15 to 18 years	1.3 mg.
Females 19 to 22 years	1.3 mg.
Females 23 to 50 years	1.2 mg.
Females 51 years and over	1.2 mg.
Pregnant women	*add* 0.3 mg.
Breast-feeding women	*add* 0.5 mg.

Greater amounts of vitamin may be needed in:
* Persons with diseases of the liver or gall bladder
* Persons who regularly drink alcohol

Symptoms of deficiency:
    Cracking of the lips
    Inflammation of the mouth, lips, or tongue
    Skin rash
    Tingling or numbness of the hands or feet

Some dietary sources:

Beans

Eggs

Fish

Green, leafy
vegetables

Liver

Whole-grain bread and
flour

Unproven uses:

Treatment or prevention of

Acne

Blood disorders

"Burning feet"
syndrome

Cataracts

Headache

Muscle cramps

Visual problems

Side effects

No side effects have been reported with the oral use of
riboflavin.

Vitamin B₃

Vitamin B_3, more commonly known as niacin or nicotinic acid, is not an innocuous substance. Niacin can produce severe, uncomfortable flushing of the skin and should
never be given as a nutritional supplement to people with
active peptic ulcers or severe low blood pressure or diabetes. Niacin is associated with a long list of side effects,
many of which are included in the table that follows.

Niacin is a "borderline" vitamin in the sense that adults
can internally produce most of their total daily requirement themselves. This plus the fact that niacin is readily
available in common foods makes niacin deficiency disease a rarity.

Niacin was involved in one of the earliest attempts at
megadose vitamin therapy. Canadian psychiatrist Abram
Hoffer noted in the 1950s that some people with pellagra,
a severe niacin deficiency state, suffered from psychosis.
When their diets were supplemented with large doses of
niacin, the psychosis improved.

Encouraged by these results, Hoffer postulated that
schizophrenia, which is characterized by psychosis, might
also improve with niacin therapy. He eventually developed

a treatment protocol that called for massive amounts of niacin to be given to schizophrenics each day. To his delight, many of them recovered.

Hoffer proclaimed his success to the world and soon psychiatrists all over North America were giving toxic doses of niacin to their schizophrenic patients. But some of them noticed that their patients didn't seem to do as well as those Hoffer described. In fact, they didn't seem to do as well as those who were given conventional medications.

What was the problem? While Hoffer continued to report good results with his patients, other psychiatrists couldn't duplicate his success.

One of the problems is that about one-third of schizophrenics improve without any treatment at all. Hoffer steadfastly refused to conduct experiments that incorporated methods intended to eliminate bias and placebo effect. When the Canadian Psychiatric Association sponsored a series of extensive and expensive evaluations of niacin in schizophrenia they found that the vitamin had no effect at all for this illness.

Vitamin B₃

Other names:
  Niacin
  Nicotinic acid
Proven functions:
  Metabolism of fats, carbohydrates, and amino acids
  High doses lower blood levels of triglycerides and cholesterol.
Recommended Dietary Allowance (1980):

Infants up to 6 months	6 mg.
Infants 6 months to 1 year	8 mg.
Children 1 to 3 years	9 mg.
Children 4 to 6 years	11 mg.
Children 7 to 10 years	16 mg.
Males 11 to 14 years	18 mg.
Males 15 to 18 years	18 mg.

Males 19 to 22 years	19 mg.
Males 23 to 50 years	18 mg.
Males 51 years and over	16 mg.
Females 11 to 14 years	15 mg.
Females 15 to 18 years	14 mg.
Females 19 to 22 years	14 mg.
Females 23 to 50 years	13 mg.
Females 51 years and over	13 mg.
Pregnant women	*add* 2 mg.
Breast-feeding women	*add* 5 mg.

Greater amounts of vitamin may be needed:

- During acute illnesses
- During periods of drastically increased exercise or physical activity
- During recovery from severe injuries or infections
- If tryptophan intake is low
- In patients taking the anti-tuberculosis drug isoniazid (Nydrazid)
- When the daily diet is abruptly increased

Symptoms of deficiency:

Confusion	Psychiatric
Diarrhea	disturbances
Drying and cracking	Reddening of the skin
of the skin	Stomach pain
Inflammation of the	Thickening of the skin
mouth and/or tongue	

Some dietary sources:

Beans	Liver
Chicken	Peas
Enriched bread or	Red meat
flour	Whole-wheat bread or
Fish	flour

Unproven uses:

Treatment or prevention of

Acne	Migraine headache
Arthritis	Motion sickness

Hardening of the arteries	Schizophrenia
	Skin rashes
Leprosy	

Side effects:

Changes in heart rate and rhythm	Intense itching
	Intense skin flushing
Diarrhea	Liver damage
Drop in blood pressure	Nausea and vomiting
Fainting	Skin rashes
Heartburn	Stomach pain
Increased blood sugar	Yellow jaundice

Niacin may worsen:

Allergic conditions	Gall bladder disease
Asthma	Gout
Bleeding disorders	Liver disease
Coronary artery disease	Peptic ulcers
Diabetes	

Vitamin B₆

Vitamin B$_6$, pyridoxine, occupies an essential role in protein metabolism. Interestingly, the requirements for this vitamin are so low it is almost impossible to induce pyridoxine deficiency by dietary restriction alone. Most cases of vitamin B$_6$ deficiency are caused by the drugs listed in the table below.

Pyridoxine has attracted attention lately because of its purported role in preventing or treating premenstrual syndrome (PMS). Unfortunately, some tests of pyridoxine in this disorder have indicated that vitamin therapy is not effective.

Pyridoxine provides an interesting example of misconceptions about vitamins. For the most part, water-soluble vitamins are not stored in the body. Because our diets normally provide excess amounts of these nutrients, the human body has never needed to develop a storage mechanism. Since we do not need to store these vitamins, we eliminate excess quantities through the urine.

For many years we have assumed that there is no such

thing as water-soluble vitamin toxicity, since the body rids itself of the superfluous materials. More recently, we have learned that this is not true.

Several cases reported in the *New England Journal of Medicine* illustrate that pyridoxine can indeed cause problems. And some of the symptoms of long-term pyridoxine toxicity are remarkably similar to the symptoms of pyridoxine deficiency!

As megadose vitamin therapies become more and more common, we may start to see more cases of vitamin toxicity—toxicities that we never knew existed.

Vitamin B₆

Other Names:
  Pyridoxal
  Pyridoxamine
  Pyridoxine
Proven functions:
  Essential for protein metabolism
Recommended Dietary Allowance (1980):

Infants up to 6 months	0.3 mg.
Infants 6 months to 1 year	0.6 mg.
Children 1 to 3 years	0.9 mg.
Children 4 to 6 years	1.3 mg.
Children 7 to 10 years	1.6 mg.
Males 11 to 14 years	1.8 mg.
Males 15 to 18 years	2.1 mg.
Males 19 to 22 years	2.2 mg.
Males 23 to 50 years	2.2 mg.
Males 51 years and over	2.2 mg.
Females 11 to 14 years	1.8 mg.
Females 15 to 18 years	2.0 mg.
Females 19 to 22 years	2.0 mg.
Females 23 to 50 years	2.0 mg.
Females 51 years and over	2.0 mg.
Pregnant women	*add* 0.6 mg.
Breast-feeding women	*add* 0.5 mg.

Greater amounts of vitamin B_6 may be needed in persons taking the following drugs:

Alcohol	Penicillamine
Ethosuximide	(Cupramine)
(Zarontin)	Phenytoin (Dilantin)
Hydralazine	Pyrazinamide
(Apresoline)	
Isoniazid (Nydrazid)	
Oral contraceptives	

Symptoms of deficiency:

Confusion	Numbness or tingling
Convulsions in infants	in the hands and/or
Depression	feet
Irritability	

Some dietary sources:

Avocados	Lima beans
Bananas	Nuts
Cabbage	Red meats
Eggs	Sweet potatoes
Fish	Whole-grain bread and
Lentils	flour

Unproven uses:

Treatment or prevention of

Asthma	Nerve disorders
Convulsions	Premenstral syndrome
Kidney stones	Psychiatric illness
Loss of appetite	Skin diseases
Nausea and vomiting, including motion sickness and morning sickness during pregnancy	

Short-term side effects of high doses:
Altered liver function
Decreases in the hormone prolactin

Long-term side effects of high doses:
Convulsions
Decreased reflexes
Progressive loss of muscle coordination and loss of sensations in the arms and legs

Vitamin B$_{12}$

The most common misuse of vitamin B$_{12}$ is as a stimulant. Cyanocobalamin, the most common form of B$_{12}$, is bright red and makes a great placebo injection. In fact, at one time it was so commonly used for this purpose that some insurance companies refused to pay for the treatments unless the doctor provided proof that the patient had a vitamin deficiency disease.

We easily obtain our daily B$_{12}$ requirements in our regular diet; there is no need to take extra. In fact, many multiple vitamin products don't contain B$_{12}$. One reason for this omission is that people who are deficient in B$_{12}$ can't absorb it from their gastrointestinal tracts, no matter how much they take.

Pernicious anemia occurs when the bone marrow can't get enough vitamin B$_{12}$. In this form of anemia the blood count drops and the red blood cells are bloated and misshapen. This vitamin deficit also causes a deterioration of nerve cells that can have crippling effects. But the disease is not due to lack of B$_{12}$ in the diet; it's due to the lack of intrinsic factor in the stomach.

Intrinsic factor is a substance formed in the liver and secreted into the stomach. Without it, vitamin B$_{12}$ cannot be absorbed, no matter how much vitamin is in the diet. Before the development of B$_{12}$ injections, the only treatment for this condition was to eat raw liver.

Today the treatment for this condition is a monthly injection of a low dose of vitamin B$_{12}$. When a person with pernicious anemia starts getting these injections, he or she feels more energetic, not because B$_{12}$ is a stimulant, but because it controls the disease that caused the fatigue.

Vitamin B$_{12}$

Other names:
    Cyanocobalamin
    Hydroxocobalamin
Proven functions:
    Necessary for maintaining nerve cells

Necessary for storage and utilization of folic acid
Necessary for the metabolism of fats
Participates in cell division

Recommended Dietary Allowance (1980):

Infants up to 6 months	0.5 mcg.
Infants 6 months to 1 year	1.5 mcg.
Children 1 to 3 years	2.0 mcg.
Children 4 to 6 years	2.5 mcg.
Children 7 to 10 years	3.0 mcg.
Males 11 to 14 years	3.0 mcg.
Males 15 to 18 years	3.0 mcg.
Males 19 to 22 years	3.0 mcg.
Males 23 to 50 years	3.0 mcg.
Males 51 years and over	3.0 mcg.
Females 11 to 14 years	3.0 mcg.
Females 15 to 18 years	3.0 mcg.
Females 19 to 22 years	3.0 mcg.
Females 23 to 50 years	3.0 mcg.
Females 51 years and over	3.0 mcg.
Pregnant women	*add* 1.0 mcg.
Breast-feeding women	*add* 1.0 mcg.

Greater amounts of vitamin may be needed in persons
taking the following drugs:

- Antiseizure medications
- Cholestyramine (Questran)
- Oral contraceptives

Symptoms of deficiency:

Anemia
Jaundice
Numbness or tingling
   in the fingers and/or
   toes

Psychiatric
   disturbances
Spastic muscle
   movements
Weakness
Weight loss

Some dietary sources:

Eggs
Fish
Liver

Milk
Red meat

Unproven uses:
Treatment or prevention of

Aging	Nerve pain
Hepatitis	Psychiatric problems
Memory loss	Sterility
Lack of appetite	Thyroid disease
Lack of energy	

Side effects:
No side effects have been reported with oral doses.

Vitamin C

Ascorbic acid, vitamin C, is the most extensively studied of all the vitamins. It is also the most misused and misunderstood of all the vitamins.

Vitamin C is a favorite of the megavitamin fanatics. They maintain that the RDA for vitamin C is totally inappropriate for your real needs, and that the only way to protect your health is to follow their unsubstantiated advice and take all the vitamin C you can gulp.

The 1980 RDA for vitamin C is a remarkably low 60 milligrams per day for adults. This intake assures that you will not develop vitamin C deficiency as long as you are in reasonably good health. Only 10 milligrams per day is required to prevent scurvy, the major complication of vitamin C deficiency.

A funny thing happens when you start to overdo it on vitamin C. Your gastrointestinal tract rejects the excess, and it doesn't get into your blood.

Although small amounts of vitamin C are normally well absorbed from the intestinal tract, it has been proven that only 50 percent of a 1500-milligram dose is absorbed. If you up the ante to 12,000 milligrams, a dose often recommended by Linus Pauling, the leading proponent of vitamin C megadoses, you only absorb 16 percent of the dose.

High doses of vitamin C are associated with gastrointestinal upset, including nausea, diarrhea, and abdominal cramps. Does this sound as if your body is telling you something?

Let's look at this another way.

A group of British physicians tested the relationship between vitamin C intake and the amount of vitamin C that made it to the bloodstream of a group of elderly women. They found that the body rapidly eliminated excess amounts of vitamin C, and this occurred much faster than they previously had imagined. In fact, they found that a sixteen-fold increase in daily vitamin C intake resulted in only a 30 percent increase of vitamin C in the blood!

An exceptionally poor way of giving vitamin C is to give your kids vitamin C chewable tablets. I had a friend who used to pass these out like candy. The problem is that vitamin C is really ascorbic *acid*, and ascorbic acid can gradually destroy the enamel on the kids' teeth. It isn't a good idea to make this or any other vitamin or medication too available to children.

High doses of vitamin C taken during pregnancy have also been implicated in causing scurvy in newborns. It appears that the excess vitamin circulating through fetal blood may alter fetal liver enzymes so that vitamin C is destroyed rapidly as a self-protective measure. When the baby is born and vitamin C intake returns to normal, the baby's liver continues to destroy vitamin C at an accelerated rate and the infant is at risk of developing scurvy.

If the drug—and at these doses vitamin C is a drug—is capable of causing these problems, what are the benefits of taking massive doses?

One of the supposed benefits is the treatment of cancer. As far as I know, the role, if there is any, of vitamin C in preventing cancer has not been properly evaluated. Studies sponsored by the National Cancer Institute and performed at the Mayo Clinic have failed to demonstrate any effect of high doses of ascorbic acid on cancerous tumors.

Vitamin C and the Common Cold—An Overrated Connection

The other purported use of megadose vitamin C, and the most controversial one, involves the common cold.

First, the good news: Vitamin C reduces the severity of the cold.

Now the bad news: That's all it does, and it doesn't do a very good job of that.

Linus Pauling has been a proponent of astronomical doses of vitamin C for years, and his theories have been put to the test at least twenty times. Unfortunately, they haven't tested well.

It appears that any slight beneficial effect that may be gained from ascorbic acid may occur with doses as low as 80 milligrams per day. That's right, a dose only 20 milligrams higher than the adult RDA! And at that dose, side effects from vitamin C are practically unheard of.

But before we get too carried away, let's look at the beneficial effects that the vitamin has.

Vitamin C has not been proven to prevent colds; it only decreases their severity slightly. And the operative word here is *slightly*. The few controlled studies that showed any benefit at all were not convincing.

Is it worth taking 10,000 to 20,000 milligrams of vitamin C a day to prevent something that may not happen at all and risk the side effects of that dose?

No way!

Is it worth taking 80 milligrams of vitamin C per day in the hopes that any cold that may occur will be a little milder?

That's up to you.

The effects of vitamin C on the common cold are so trivial that I don't bother to take it myself. In fact, we don't even have any vitamin C supplements in our house.

Don't put too much faith in vitamin C if you develop a cold. Go back and read the information in chapter 2.

===

Vitamin C

Other names:
   Antiscorbutic vitamin
   Ascorbic acid
Proven functions:
   Assists in the biosynthesis of neurotransmitters
   Assists in the formation of collagen tissue
   Facilitates absorption of iron from the intestine
   Necessary for the utilization of iron
   Necessary to convert folic acid to its active form
   Helps to preserve blood vessel function

Recommended Dietary Allowance (1980):

Infants up to 6 months	35 mg.
Infants 6 months to 1 year	35 mg.
Children 1 to 3 years	45 mg.
Children 4 to 6 years	45 mg.
Children 7 to 10 years	45 mg.
Males 11 to 14 years	50 mg.
Males 15 to 18 years	60 mg.
Males 19 to 22 years	60 mg.
Males 23 to 50 years	60 mg.
Males 51 years and over	60 mg.
Females 11 to 14 years	50 mg.
Females 15 to 18 years	60 mg.
Females 19 to 22 years	60 mg.
Females 23 to 50 years	60 mg.
Females 51 years and over	60 mg.
Pregnant women	*add* 20 mg.
Breast-feeding women	*add* 40 mg.

Greater amounts of vitamin may be needed in:

- Breast-feeding
- Cancer
- Chronic diarrhea
- Cigarette smoking
- Peptic ulcers
- Pregnancy
- Recovery from surgery
- Severe burns
- Thyroid disease

Symptoms of deficiency:

Bleeding beneath the skin
Bleeding from the gums
Bleeding into muscles and joints

Dental disease
Psychiatric disorders
Tiredness

Some dietary sources:

Cauliflower
Citrus fruits
Green vegetables
Leafy vegetables
Melons

Papaya
Rose hips
Strawberries
Tomatoes

Unproven uses:
  Treatment or prevention of
  Acne
  Allergies
  Anemia
  Bedsores
  Bleeding disorders
  Blood clots
  Bone fractures
  Cancer
  Complications of
    diabetes
  Crib death
  Dental disease
  Diarrhea
  Eye diseases

  Fatigue
  Hardening of the
    arteries
  Heat Prostration
  Infection
  Infertility, sterility, or
    impotence
  Lowering cholesterol
  Lung disease caused
    by smoking
  Peptic ulcer
  Psychiatric illness in
    the absence of a
    deficiency state
  Stress

Side effects:
  Abdominal cramps
  Decreased absorption of vitamin B_{12}
  Destruction of red blood cells
  Diarrhea
  Interference with tests for sugar in the urine and for
    blood in stool or urine
  Kidney stones
  Nausea
  Rebound scurvy in infants
  Sickle cell crisis

Oil-Soluble Vitamins

The oil-soluble vitamins are just as important to the normal function of your body as the water-soluble vitamins. There is, however, one significant difference between them. While the water-soluble vitamins may be overused, misused, and abused, their toxicities are trivial compared to their oil-soluble cousins.

The major difference between the water-soluble vitamins and the oil-solubles is that the body stores only small quantities of the water-solubles and eliminates the excess.

They, therefore, have relatively little risk of toxicity. The oil-soluble vitamins, on the other hand, may be stored in considerable quantities in the body's fat and oil tissues. This storage ability can change an essential nutrient to a lethal toxin.

Vitamin A

Vitamin A is a collective term that applies to three major biochemicals: retinol, retinal, and retinoic acid. Some of the characteristics of this vitamin are listed in the table that follows.

Vitamin A is essential for proper skin formation and function as well as nerve activity. It is also necessary for vision. Deficiencies may cause night blindness and drying of the conjunctiva on the eye surface. However, there is no proof that vitamin A in normal or megadoses has any effect on any eye condition other than those caused by vitamin A deficiency.

Moderation is the key to dealing with vitamin A and the other oil-soluble vitamins. The first reports of vitamin A toxicity occurred in 1857 when Arctic hunters became sick from eating polar bear livers, which are extremely high in vitamin A content.

Today the dangers of vitamin A toxicity are widely known and discussed on television and other media. Ironically, we also see more cases of vitamin A toxicity than ever before, especially in children whose parents are trying to use vitamin supplements to keep them healthy.

One of the problems with vitamin A toxicity is its insidious onset. Daily doses above 50,000 micrograms will cause symptoms of poisoning in an adult in about a year. Unfortunately, the delay in the onset of toxicity obscures the cause of illness. Even then, the early symptoms (see the table below) are vague and can be mistaken for other problems, leading to a delay in diagnosis and proper treatment.

Further confusing the issue are the claims that vitamin E can protect the body from vitamin A toxicity. It appears that dosing with vitamin E can lower the levels of vitamin A circulating in the blood. However, recent studies indicate that this effect results in larger amounts of vitamin A entering body tissues, causing an actual *increase* in vitamin A toxicity.

Since there is no good reason to use vitamins A and E together in large doses, why run the risk of toxicity with either one? .

Probably the most insidious side effect of vitamin A is its tendency to cause birth defects in children of women who take higher than recommended doses during pregnancy, especially in the first eight weeks of pregnancy. Vitamin A has been associated with bone problems, stunted infant growth, and other birth defects. At present it appears that it is not safe for pregnant women to take more than 1800 micrograms of retinol per day. The RDA for vitamin A for a pregnant woman is only 1000 micrograms per day.

How much vitamin A should you take to supplement your regular diet?

Usually none. A halfway decent diet provides more than enough vitamin A. For example, a single four-ounce serving of liver supplies enough vitamin A for a week. Even if you aren't a liver lover, you can get plenty of vitamin A in fish, eggs, and dairy products. In addition, your body is able to produce some of its own vitamin A from carotene, an orange pigment found in carrots and some other vegetables.

Due to the abundance of vitamin A in the diet, as well as the body's ability to take care of some of its own needs, vitamin A deficiency is rare in developed countries. More cases of vitamin A deficiency are caused by intestinal malabsorption diseases than by malnutrition.

Vitamin A for Acne and Cancer Prevention?

Vitamin A proponents now claim two uses for megadoses of vitamin A: treatment of acne and prevention of cancer.

Vitamin A was first described as an acne treatment in 1943. Since then it has been said to be the panacea for a wide variety of skin diseases. Unfortunately, you would have to take toxic doses of vitamin A for it to have even a small effect on acne. The good news, however, is that chemists have been able to build vitamin A-like molecules that are effective for acne with less risk of toxicity. These drugs are restricted to prescription-only status, but most physicians are very familiar with their use as well as the types of acne that respond best to them.

Vitamin A may be effective in preventing some types of cancer, particularly in smokers. Unfortunately, some preliminary but not confirmed encouraging reports have been cited by some vitamin proponents as proof of the vitamin's anticancer effect.

It appears that large daily doses of vitamin A may prevent some cases of cancer of the lung, bladder, and throat in a small percentage of the population. The kicker is that you have to poison yourself with the vitamin to prevent the cancer. In other words, you might try to prevent a cancer you may never get by taking doses of a vitamin that cause intolerable side effects, even death.

In the meantime, chemists are looking for less toxic vitamin analogs that might have the same or a better effect in cancer prevention. But you don't have to sit back and wait for them to come up with a miracle substance. Vitamins aren't the total answer to a healthy life. For example, it's ridiculous to smoke a pack of cigarettes a day and then try to prevent lung cancer by taking a vitamin. If you really want to prevent cancer and other diseases, improve your life-style. No vitamin can substitute for a decent diet, regular hours, routine exercise, and avoidance of known health risks.

Vitamin A

Other names or constituents:
  Beta-carotene
  Retinal
  Retinoic acid
  Retinol
  Retinyl acetate
Proven functions:
  Essential to vision
  Maintains cell membranes

Necessary for growth
Necessary for function of the immune system
Necessary for sexual function and fertility
Stimulates cell growth

Recommended Dietary Allowance (1980):

Infants up to 6 months	420 mcg.
Infants 6 months to 1 year	400 mcg.
Children 1 to 3 years	400 mcg.
Children 4 to 6 years	500 mcg.
Children 7 to 10 years	700 mcg.
Males 11 to 14 years	1000 mcg.
Males 15 to 18 years	1000 mcg.
Males 19 to 22 years	1000 mcg.
Males 23 to 50 years	1000 mcg.
Males 51 years and over	1000 mcg.
Females 11 to 14 years	800 mcg.
Females 15 to 18 years	800 mcg.
Females 19 to 22 years	800 mcg.
Females 23 to 50 years	800 mcg.
Females 51 years and over	800 mcg.
Pregnant women	*add* 200 mcg.
Breast-feeding women	*add* 400 mcg.

Greater amounts of vitamin may be needed in:

- Persons taking the following drugs:
  Cholestyramine (Questran)
  Mineral oil
  Spironolactone
- Bladder infection
- Cancer
- Cirrhosis of the liver
- Cystic fibrosis
- Jaundice
- Kidney infection
- Malabsorption syndrome
- Pneumonia
- Prostate disease
- Tuberculosis

Symptoms of deficiency:

Altered tooth formation
Birth defects
Decreased resistance to infection
Impaired nerve function
Intolerance to sunlight
Night blindness
Reduced bone formation
Reduced tear production

Some dietary sources:

Butter
Carrots
Cheese
Crabmeat
Cream
Eggs
Fish

Fish liver oil,
  especially cod
Fortified margarine
Liver
Milk
Sweet potatoes

Unproven uses:

Treatment or prevention of
Bone disease
Cancer
Dental disease

Infections
Poor vision
Skin diseases

Short-term side effects of high doses:

Birth defects
Bleeding under or into
  the skin
Bone pain
Cracking of the lips
Dizziness
Drowsiness
Elevated blood
  calcium
  concentration
Enlargement of the
  liver or spleen

Fluid retention and
  swelling
Hair loss
Headache due to
  increased pressure
  on the brain
Nausea
Skin peeling
Vomiting

Long-term side effects of high doses:

Anemia
Arthritis-like bone or
  joint pain
Birth defects
Bleeding disorders
Bone deterioration
Brittle nails
Double vision
Enlargement of the
  liver and spleen
Fever
Hair loss and impaired
  hair regrowth
Headache

Inflamed mouth,
  tongue, and lips
Insomnia
Irritability
Itching
Jaundice
Loss of appetite
Muscle soreness
Nosebleed
Reddened, peeling,
  and itching skin
Sweating
Weight loss

Vitamin D

Like vitamin A, vitamin D is a collection of several similar chemical substances. This vitamin is required for the proper absorption and disposition of calcium in the body.

Vitamin D is also similar to vitamin A in that the body can form significant amounts of the vitamin from available materials. Exposure of the skin to sunlight causes cholesterol to form a substance very similar to vitamin D. This substance circulates through blood until it reaches the kidneys, where it is "activated," forming true vitamin D. If you have kidney disease, your doctor may need to prescribe special forms of vitamin D to prevent a deficiency disease.

Your dietary vitamin D requirements depend upon the amount of sun exposure you get or don't get.

You don't need to get your vitamin D out of a pill bottle. Even if you live in a cave and never see the sun, you can get all the vitamin D you need from as little as a quart of vitamin-enriched milk a day.

Vitamin D shares one other characteristic with vitamin A, and even goes it one better. Vitamin D is the most toxic of all the vitamins. Children are at greatest risk of toxicity, usually because parents believe they have to pour vitamins down kids' throats to keep them healthy.

Don't give your children vitamin D supplements unless your doctor advises it. The same advice applies to adults.

Vitamin D causes problems by rearranging the calcium in your body. Vitamin D normally plucks calcium out of the food in your intestine and facilitates its transfer across the intestinal wall and into the blood. From there, vitamin D regulates the amount of calcium that goes into and comes out of your bones. If you're carrying a proper amount of vitamin D in your body, the system works pretty well.

But if you have too much vitamin D on board you're in deep trouble. Vitamin D continues to absorb calcium from the intestine. The more vitamin D there is, the more calcium that is absorbed. Once the calcium is in the blood, vitamin D has to find a place for it. If the bones are full, vitamin D starts stashing calcium wherever it can find a place, including the heart, liver, and kidneys. Vitamin D toxicity and the accompanying calcium overload can lead to kidney failure and heart attacks in adults, and mental retardation and stunted growth in children.

Vitamin D

Other names or constituents:
Calcifediol
Calcitriol
Cholecalciferol
Dihydrotachysterol
Ergocalciferol

Proven functions:
Bone dissolution
Bone growth
Incorporation of
    calcium into bone
Intestinal absorption of
    calcium

Recommended Dietary Allowance (1980):

Infants up to 6 months	10 mcg.
Infants 6 months to 1 year	10 mcg.
Children 1 to 3 years	10 mcg.
Children 4 to 6 years	10 mcg.
Children 7 to 10 years	10 mcg.
Males 11 to 14 years	10 mcg.
Males 15 to 18 years	10 mcg.
Males 19 to 22 years	7.5 mcg.
Males 23 to 50 years	5 mcg.
Males 51 years and over	5 mcg.
Females 11 to 14 years	10 mcg.
Females 15 to 18 years	10 mcg.
Females 19 to 22 years	7.5 mcg.
Females 23 to 50 years	5 mcg.
Females 51 years and over	5 mcg.
Pregnant women	*add* 5 mcg.
Breast-feeding women	*add* 5 mcg.

Greater amounts of vitamin may be needed in:

Persons taking the following drugs:
Anticonvulsants

Phosphate-containing drugs, such as antacids and laxatives
- Lack of sun exposure
- Low-fat or fat-free diets
- Malabsorption syndrome

Symptoms of deficiency:

Bloated belly
Dental cavities
Difficulty walking or climbing stairs
Frequent bone fractures
Nervousness
Pain in the legs and back

Pigeon breast
Poor muscle development
Softening of bone
Spinal curvature
Tooth malformation

Some dietary sources:

Butter
Cheese
Eggs
Fish liver oil, especially cod

Fortified margarine
Fortified milk

Unproven uses:

Treatment or prevention of
Colds

Eye infections

Side effects:

Abnormal heart rhythms
Arrested growth in children
Birth defects
Burning or inflamed eyes
Constipation
Decreased sex drive
Dry mouth
Fever in children
Hardening of the arteries
Headache
Hearing loss
High blood pressure

Increased blood cholesterol
Increased urination
Itching
Kidney failure
Kidney stones
Lack of appetite
Mental retardation
Metallic taste in the mouth
Muscle aches and stiffness
Nausea
Osteoporosis (weakening of bone)
Thirst

Vomiting
Weight loss

Vitamin E

Next to vitamin C, vitamin E has to be the most over-promoted and overrated of all the vitamins.

Vitamin E has been promoted for a wide variety of mild and not so mild illnesses. Unfortunately, proof of the vitamin's efficacy for almost all of these claims is nonexistent. Nevertheless, people seem to be unwilling to accept the fact that vitamin E has no effect on the illnesses that plague mankind.

Vitamin E is necessary for life, but beyond that its exact function is unclear. Vitamin E deficiencies are seen in newborn babies who have a rare type of anemia. In adults vitamin E deficits are only seen in connection with intestinal malabsorption problems, and even then there are seldom any symptoms of illness.

Vitamin E may provide some benefit to people with a condition called intermittent claudication, a disease where circulation in the legs decreases with exercise. Canadian researchers found that people with this condition could walk farther without pain following doses of vitamin E. However, current prescription drug therapy is more effective and reliable. Those who use the vitamin for this purpose should also be aware that vitamin E does not stop or even slow the progress of the disease; it only temporarily relieves some of the symptoms.

Vitamin E has also been investigated for a possible role in treating or preventing coronary artery disease, the condition that often leads to angina and heart attacks. Two well-controlled studies failed to find any significant benefit as a result of taking the vitamin.

The table below lists both proven and unproven uses of vitamin E. The truth of the matter is that vitamin E is much more important to animals than it is to humans. Some of the unproven uses of the vitamin, such as improved fertility and sexual function, relate only to rats, not humans.

One reason vitamin E deficiency is rare is that the vitamin is found in so many different food groups. Tocopherols, the chemical constituents of vitamin E, are found in significant quantities in grain, fish, vegetables, and eggs. The body also stores tocopherol efficiently, so that once the vitamin is absorbed, it can be saved until it is needed.

Vitamin E is remarkable among the oil-soluble vitamins in that it is relatively nontoxic. One experiment demonstrated that people can take up to 800 milligrams (or International Units) per day for a period of three years without serious side effects.

But that is not to say that vitamin E is free of side effects. Megadoses, doses ten or more times higher than the RDA, are associated with headaches, nausea, blurred vision, chapped lips, and the other side effects listed in the table.

The bottom line on vitamin E is that it probably won't hurt you to take a small dose each day, but it won't do you much good, either. If you insist on taking any drug or vitamin that you don't need, you run the risk of unnecessary side effects. I don't take vitamin E, and I don't advise it for you without your doctor's approval.

Vitamin E

Other names or constituents:
Tocopherol
Proven functions:
Improves blood flow to the legs
Necessary for drug-metabolizing enzymes
Necessary for nerve and muscle function
Stabilizes cell membranes
Synthesis of blood proteins
Recommended Dietary Allowance (1980):
1 milligram (mg.) equals approximately 1 International Unit (I.U.)

Infants up to 6 months	3 mg.
Infants 6 months to 1 year	4 mg.
Children 1 to 3 years	5 mg.
Children 4 to 6 years	6 mg.

Children 7 to 10 years	7 mg.
Males 11 to 14 years	8 mg.
Males 15 to 18 years	10 mg.
Males 19 to 22 years	10 mg.
Males 23 to 50 years	10 mg.
Males 51 years and over	10 mg.
Females 11 to 14 years	8 mg.
Females 15 to 18 years	8 mg.
Females 19 to 22 years	8 mg.
Females 23 to 50 years	8 mg.
Females 51 years and over	8 mg.
Pregnant women	*add* 2 mg.
Breast-feeding women	*add* 3 mg.

Greater amounts of vitamin may be needed in:

- Increased dietary fat consumption
- Low birth-weight infants

Symptoms of deficiency:
Degeneration of the retina of the eye
Destruction of red blood cells in infants
Muscle incoordination

Some dietary sources:

Dairy products	Nuts
Eggs	Red meat
Fish	Vegetable oils
Green vegetables	Whole-grain flour or bread

Unproven uses:
Treatment or prevention of

Aging	Burns
Anemia	Cancer
Arthritis	Diabetes
Baldness	Fatigue
Breast cysts	Frostbite
Heart disease	Peptic ulcers
Infertility	Sexual problems
Jaundice	Sickle cell anemia
Leg cramps	Skin problems
Liver disease	Smog-related breathing problems

Menopause-related
  problems
Miscarriage
Muscular dystrophy
Side effects:
  Blood clots
  Blurred vision
  Diarrhea
  Dizziness
  Drowsiness
  Inflammation of the
    mouth and lips
  Increased blood
    cholesterol levels

Nerve disorders
Thyroid disease
Vitamin A toxicity
Warts

Nausea
Skin rash
Stomach cramps
Vomiting
Headache
Weakness

Mineral Supplements

Minerals are just as important to health as vitamins and are probably just as misunderstood.

Minerals are essential nutrients that perform several vital functions. They strengthen bones and teeth, they maintain the form and function of cells, they assist in regulating the fluid balance of the body, and they are incorporated into enzymes and other proteins.

All minerals can be obtained in sufficient amounts from food sources, but unlike the vitamins, the amounts of minerals in plant food sources fluctuate depending upon the composition of the soil in which they are grown. For instance, the iron content of spinach will vary according to the amount of iron in the farmer's field.

Most people are able to get all of their mineral requirements from diet alone, but mineral deficiencies may become a more significant problem as our society continues to use more and more processed foods. There seem to be dozens of different types and combinations of minerals on pharmacy and health food shelves, but we will concern ourselves only with the three most popular ones—calcium, iron, and zinc.

Calcium

The teeth and bones contain 99 percent of the body's calcium. The remainder is needed for enzyme functions, muscle contractions (including the heart), and blood coagulation. The bones act as the body's calcium storehouse. When calcium is needed elsewhere in the body, vitamin D pulls calcium out of bone to make it available for other functions.

Calcium provides strength to bones. Lack or loss of calcium in children may lead to bone-softening diseases like rickets and osteomalacia. In adults osteoporosis, a loss of bone tissue, is more of a problem.

Osteoporosis—A Threat to the Elderly

Osteoporosis is the great crippler of the elderly. As we age we absorb less and less calcium from our daily diet. While this is a problem for elderly men, the problem is critical for postmenopausal women.

The female hormone estrogen normally assists in depositing calcium into bone, but at menopause the amounts of estrogen that women produce fall precipitously. While this isn't a problem right away, it becomes one with time. After menopause, women lose almost 1 percent of their bone mass each year.

Father Time takes his toll on the bones as they become less and less calcified. Finally the bones reach the point where they break easily and repair slowly. Orthopedic surgeons estimate that 90 percent of broken bones in people over the age of sixty are due to osteoporosis.

There are effective treatments for osteoporosis if they are started early enough. Your doctor can prescribe hormones or fluoride supplements. Or you can buy nonprescription calcium and vitamin D products. But before you do, you should know some of the limits and hazards of self-treatment.

The major limitation to using calcium to treat or prevent osteoporosis is that we don't know if it works. While it is prudent to make sure you get 1200 milligrams of calcium per day, calcium supplements have never been proven to have a beneficial effect on aging bones. We can only hope that scientists will be able to confirm this effect in the near future.

Many calcium supplements contain a small amount of vitamin D. The reason for this is that vitamin D is necessary for the intestinal absorption of calcium, and a little extra vitamin D should help you absorb more calcium than you normally would.

Vitamin D has another function. It distributes calcium around the body for its non-bone-forming functions. And where does it get the calcium to do this? It takes it *out of* bone! Ironically, too much vitamin D can actually make your bone condition worse.

But what about plain calcium? Can't you just take a megadose of calcium to make sure you're getting enough?

The Food and Nutrition Board said in its 1980 RDA that a postmenopausal woman needs a total of 800 milligrams of calcium per day from all sources. Others maintain that if you are in this group you should take between 1200 and 1500 milligrams of calcium daily. These levels may prevent, or at least slow down, age-related bone destruction. But what happens if you overdo it?

There is some evidence that daily calcium doses in excess of 1500 milligrams, and certainly over 2000 milligrams, may actually *decrease* the amount of calcium that is incorporated into your bones. While you may think you are taking good care of yourself, you may actually be damaging your bone structure.

In any event, *don't try to self-treat osteoporosis*. Not all postmenopausal women need calcium supplements, and most women will never develop osteoporosis. Let your doctor evaluate the state of your bones and determine what needs to be done. If you aggressively self-medicate, you may find yourself in more trouble than you had when you started.

Calcium Supplements—Follow Your Physician's Advice

Excess calcium can cause a wide variety of problems. Besides the effects on bone, calcium can cause irregular heartbeat, damage blood vessels, and cause kidney stones, muscle weakness and pain, fatigue, and headache.

Dairy products are the best source of calcium. Eight

ounces of milk contain about 300 milligrams and three glasses of milk per day, or its equivalent in yogurt or cheese, can supply almost all the calcium you need. If you have a weight problem or if your doctor has told you to limit your fat intake, you may be able to use skim milk as a substitute for whole milk.

If we assume for a moment that you and your doctor agree that you need a calcium supplement, which one do you choose? All calcium products aren't alike, and those that contain the highest concentrations of calcium aren't necessarily the best.

You can't buy plain calcium; it has to be part of a "salt" or chemical compound, and calcium salts vary in potency. For instance, a 1000-milligram tablet of calcium carbonate contains only 400 milligrams of "elemental" or actual calcium. That doesn't sound very good, but it's the richest source we have. The same strength tablet of calcium phosphate has 290 milligrams, while calcium lactate has 130 milligrams, and calcium gluconate contains a lowly 90 milligrams of actual calcium.

Well, that makes things a lot easier. We should pick a calcium carbonate product, shouldn't we?

Unfortunately, the richest calcium source is also one of the hardest to absorb from the intestine. While healthy adults absorb 30 to 60 percent of the calcium in the diet, these same people only absorb 8 to 24 percent of the calcium in a calcium carbonate tablet!

What happened?

In order to understand some of the complexities of calcium absorption, you have to know that the body can only absorb foods and nutrients that dissolve in water. In some cases the acids in the stomach can convert nutrients to water-soluble compounds.

What is calcium carbonate? You're probably most familiar with it as limestone, marble, or granite. Those minerals aren't very water soluble, are they?

The most common commercial source of calcium for mineral supplements is oyster shell. You've seen the ads for oyster shell products—in fact, one drug company proudly announced an $11 million advertising campaign, complete with massive couponing, network television commercials, and magazine ads, all intended to proclaim the benefits of their oyster shell calcium product. A supposed advantage of these products is that they are a "natural" source of calcium, although I can't imagaine an "unnatural" source of calcium.

Oyster shell *is* a rich source of calcium, but stop to think for a minute. If oyster shells could dissolve in water, oysters couldn't live in them.

But doesn't the stomach convert calcium carbonate to something we can use?

Yes, but the process isn't that simple. When we swallow a calcium carbonate tablet, the acid in the stomach converts some of it to calcium chloride. Calcium chloride is water-soluble and capable of being absorbed through the intestine. But the story doesn't stop there.

As calcium chloride passes through the intestinal channel, guess what happens? Most of it is converted back to calcium carbonate, and we're back where we started, with one difference. Our calcium carbonate has passed the stomach, and there is no more acid around to change it to the chloride again. Most of our calcium continues through the intestinal tract and is eliminated in the stool. Consequently, only a small percentage of the calcium carbonate, that rich source of "natural" calcium, ever gets to your bones.

To make matters worse, as we age we progressively lose the ability to form stomach acid. Researchers have been able to show that older people, who need it most, can't absorb as much calcium from calcium carbonate as younger people do.

So what's the alternative?

Unfortunately, there isn't a good alternative.

We absorb water-soluble calcium salts about twice as well as calcium carbonate, but they only have about one-fourth the calcium content of calcium carbonate.

I normally recommend calcium gluconate or lactate to people who come to me for help with their calcium supplements. These salts are better absorbed than calcium carbonate, but they are also considerably more expensive.

One source that I don't recommend at all is dolomite. Dolomite is a mineral that contains a high concentration of calcium and magnesium. It may also contain lead, mercury, and arsenic. The FDA has issued warnings about the health risks involved with regular use of dolomite. You don't need to poison yourself when there are plenty of safer calcium products on the market.

In any event, don't self-medicate with calcium without your doctor's supervision. Unnecessary or overly ambitious calcium supplementation is not only expensive, it may be detrimental to your health.

Iron

Iron deficiency is the most common mineral deficiency state in premenopausal women. Iron deficiency is caused by inadequate intake of iron, blood loss, pregnancy, malabsorption, or breast-feeding. Iron deficits seldom cause death in developed countries, but they are responsible for poor health and decreased productivity.

Iron is critical to the function of blood. The red blood cells that transport oxygen around the body cannot function without iron. Untreated iron deficiency anemia is basically a disease of slow suffocation of all parts of the body.

People with iron deficiency anemia may be pale, listless, have nausea, dizzy episodes, difficulty concentrating, loss of breath after mild exercise, and diarrhea or constipation. In more severe cases, they may have sores in the mouth, liver problems, and irregular heartbeats.

The blood of a patient with iron deficiency anemia has a characteristic appearance under a microscope. Anemic red blood cells are usually small and pale. With proper treatment, young red cells called reticulocytes appear to announce the onset of recovery from the anemic condition.

Iron deficiency anemia responds quickly to iron supplements, but *don't try self-treatment*. Your doctor needs to determine both your dose and your duration of treatment. Besides that, there are many types of anemia, some of which can be dangerous if proper treatment is delayed. Only iron deficiency anemia responds to iron supplements.

The most common cause of iron deficiency anemia is

menstrual blood loss. A woman loses two to three ounces of blood with each menstrual period. This amount of blood contains about 1.5 milligrams of iron, but that iron can be difficult to replace.

Ironically, there's more than enough iron in the diet to counterbalance the amount lost during a menstrual period. However, we are able to absorb only 5 to 10 percent of the iron we ingest.

The pharmaceutical industry hasn't let any grass grow under its feet in regard to iron supplements. There is a plethora of products promoted exclusively to women with brand names that start with Fem-something or Woman's-whatever.

Iron absorption is about as complicated as calcium absorption. Iron must be in the form of a water-soluble salt before absorption can take place. This is a bigger problem than you may think. Most vegetable sources, like spinach, contain *insoluble* iron; consequently you derive little if any benefit from eating vegetables that are rich in iron.

When a soluble iron salt is swallowed it begins to dissolve in the fluids in the digestive tract. As long as it stays in a water-soluble chemical form it is a candidate for absorption, but if it is changed to a less soluble form or binds with food, the percentage of iron absorbed is reduced.

Some experiments have shown that ascorbic acid taken with a dose of iron will help keep the iron in a soluble state. Unfortunately, the improvement in iron absorption isn't significant. You're probably wasting your time and money with vitamin C.

The most common cause of iron deficiency in men is peptic ulcer disease. This one presents a real dilemma.

People who have bleeding ulcers, even if the bleeding is only minimal, lose enough blood to develop iron deficiency anemia. It may seem that you need to take some iron to reverse the anemia, but that isn't the case.

One of the most common side effects of iron supplements is gastric irritation. This is the last thing you need if you have an ulcer. Iron supplements can worsen an ulcer or even reactivate an old one. Anyone with either anemia or a peptic ulcer should be seeing a doctor. If you have both, you shouldn't be dabbling with self-medication.

People with rheumatoid arthritis are at risk of anemia, not only because of their disease, but also as a result of their therapy. Most of the drugs used to treat arthritis, including aspirin and to a lesser extent ibuprofen, are associated with stomach irritation and blood loss. In addition, arthritics often develop anemias that don't respond to iron. Once again, self-treatment can be dangerous—see your doctor.

Iron Supplements—Use with Care

What do you eat if you want to increase your iron intake?

Unfortunately, most vegetables are out because of iron absorption problems. The only good sources of iron are animal protein, particularly liver and red meat, and iron-enriched flour and bread.

Because of the limited number of dietary sources, there is a brisk market in iron supplements. Many of these are excellent for the treatment or prevention of iron deficiency, but choose wisely. Many of the claims made for these products are overly enthusiastic.

First of all, watch out for the dose of the drug. You don't want to take the dose intended for people with anemia if you aren't anemic. And if you are anemic, get your doctor's okay before you start self-treating.

The reason you don't want to take an anemic's dose is that iron is a long-term toxin. If you take too much over a long period of time, it can cause serious problems. But we'll talk about iron toxicity a little later.

For most people the small amount of iron included in vitamin-with-iron combination products is about right. You don't have to overdo it to prevent iron deficiency.

The next consideration in choosing an iron product is the iron salt. As is the case with calcium, the iron or ferrous salt can make all the difference in the world. Ferrous citrate, tartrate, and pyrophosphate aren't absorbed as well as are ferrous sulfate, gluconate, fumarate, or ferrocholinate. Even the most soluble salts contain varying amounts of iron. Ferrous fumarate and sulfate are the richest sources, while ferrous gluconate and ferrocholinate have about half the iron content of the other two.

Iron supplements come in tablets, capsules, sustained-release tablets and capsules, and liquid forms. As a general rule, the plain tablets are the least expensive and provide the greatest degree of iron absorption. The iron in the liquid forms may attack the teeth and stain them. Sustained-release forms are the least effective.

Sustained-release products are expensive to manufacture, but they generally provide one benefit—they cause less stomach irritation than the other forms. The sustained-release products are specially formulated to dissolve only after they pass the stomach and duodenum, the areas most sensitive to iron. Unfortunately, most of them don't dissolve until they pass the portion of the small intestine that absorbs most of our iron. Consequently, sustained-release products dump most of their iron into your stool, where it doesn't do anyone any good.

Iron Toxicity—A Serious Risk

Iron is a dangerous drug. In normal doses it can cause numerous side effects, including nausea, vomiting, a bad taste in the mouth, constipation, stomach pain, and dark, tarlike stools. But these are mild compared to overdoses.

As few as five iron tablets can kill a two-year-old child. Iron should never be left within a child's reach, and if you don't need your iron tablets anymore, throw them out. Death from iron poisoning is excruciatingly painful and totally unnecessary if adequate precautions are taken. (These precautions are discussed in chapter 11.)

A less obvious problem occurs in people who take iron supplements but don't need them. Long-term iron toxicity is insidious. It can creep up on you after years of use and completely ruin your health.

The single most important feature of iron poisoning is that the body has no natural means to get rid of the overload. Most drugs are eliminated or detoxified by the kidneys or liver, but not iron. Most drugs perform their intended function and are destroyed, but not iron. Most drugs leave the body a few hours after a dose, but not iron.

The iron you absorb from a meal or from a tablet stays with you until you either bleed or your skin flakes off. The iron in red blood cells is continually recycled by one of the body's most efficient mechanisms. Since absorbable iron is so scarce in the diet, the body does everything it can to hang on to it for as long as possible.

That's the problem with taking iron you don't need. If you take unnecessary iron for long periods, it eventually saturates all of the body's storage areas. Since iron can't be excreted, it has to go somewhere else—and it does. It begins piling up in the spleen, the liver, the heart, and the pancreas. This abnormal accumulation of iron eventually poisons these organs and, if left untreated, progresses to death.

Don't take iron if you don't need it. The only groups who routinely need iron supplements are children, because they are outgrowing their iron stores, and menstruating women. *Adult men and postmenopausal women should never take iron supplements without a doctor's supervision.*

Vitamins and Minerals—What Should You Take?

Most people don't need to take any at all, but if you insist on vitamins or if you are in a high-risk group for vitamin deficiency, there are some that are safer and make more sense than others.

Which Minerals Should You Take?

Since calcium, iron and zinc deficiencies rarely occur at the same time in the same person, it doesn't make sense to use a product that contains all of them.

Nor should you self-medicate with any of them. Consult your doctor about your need for minerals. A physician can test for mineral deficiencies and can advise you on the best way to treat and prevent them.

Menstruating women are at relatively high risk of iron deficiency anemia, but not all women develop this problem. It doesn't do any good to "stock up" your body stores of iron if you don't need to. Again, your doctor can tell you if you need supplements, even the ones that are combined with multiple vitamins.

Zinc

Zinc is an enigma. It is found in a wide assortment of enzymes and can therefore be assumed to be essential to life. On the other hand, it is extremely difficult to find obvious cases of zinc deficiency.

Children who are zinc-deficient grow more slowly than other children, and adults who are deficient have slow-healing wounds and impaired taste and smell. None of these are outstanding diagnostic criteria.

As is the case with calcium and iron, giving zinc to a person who doesn't need it does no good and may do harm. Zinc supplements can return a deficient child's growth rate to normal, but zinc cannot make a nondeficient child grow faster. Zinc supplements can make a de-

---

Should You Take Vitamin Supplements?

There is a segment of the population at risk of vitamin deficiencies, and people included therein may benefit from vitamin supplements. They generally include

- People who are taking medications that eliminate vitamins faster than normal (ask your pharmacist if this affects you)
- People whose disease states or economic conditions preclude them from eating properly
- People with intestinal absorption problems (they should be under a doctor's care anyway)
- People who have increased metabolic requirements (such as those caused by pregnancy or recent surgery)

When it is time to choose a product, look for one that provides close to 100 percent of the U.S.R.D.A. for each of its ingredients. You don't need supertherapeutic formulations. Likewise, the ''geriatric'' or ''senior'' formulations usually provide much more vitamin at much more expense than you really need. I've seen too many seniors spend their limited Social Security money on high-priced vitamins that they really don't need.

ficient person's cuts and scratches heal faster, but they cannot speed healing in a nondeficient person.

An adult only needs minuscule amounts of zinc in the diet, about 15 milligrams per day. This is easily provided by beef, poultry, wheat germ, peanuts, pork, beans, eggs, and milk. Supplements are not necessary if you have an adequate diet.

The zinc supplements that are on the market are much less complicated than either calcium or iron. Zinc is usually used in either the sulfate or gluconate salts. Both are soluble in water and are absorbed well. The product label will indicate the amount of actual zinc per dose. In truth, that doesn't really matter, because you probably don't need it.

Zinc is not free of side effects. Most people have little more than a mild upset stomach from a "normal" dose, but high doses are another matter. A single 220-milligram capsule of zinc sulfate can cause intense nausea and vomiting. Higher doses can cause burning in the stomach, dizziness, sweating, and increased heart rate.

Since there is little likelihood that you need zinc, don't take it. Avoid vitamin products that seem to add it to their other ingredients as an afterthought, and certainly don't take plain zinc capsules without consulting your doctor.

The Pharmacist's Prescription for Vitamins and Minerals

Before reaching for a vitamin supplement, see if you can improve your diet by using the four major food groups. Vitamins are not a substitute for a balanced diet.

Read the labels and follow the directions on any vitamin product.

Take vitamins with meals.

Store all vitamin products out of reach of children.

Do not tell children that their vitamins are "candy."

Vitamins are not a substitute for a balanced diet.

See the Doctor if . . .
- You have any digestive disease.
- You constantly feel tired or lack energy.
- You look pale.
- Your diet is poor.
- You reach menopause.
- You drink or smoke heavily.

11

Children Are Not Little Adults

I am an old man,
but in many senses a very young man.
And this is what I want you to be,
young, young all your life, and to say
things to the world that are true.
—Pablo Casals (1876–1973)

How do children differ from adults?

They differ in terms of disease. The "childhood diseases" such as measles and chicken pox occur only rarely in adults.

They differ in response to their disease. Children seem to tolerate fever better than adults, but a two-day episode of diarrhea could be fatal to a newborn.

And they differ in terms of drug dosing. Deciding the proper dose for your child is just as important as selecting the proper drug. Unfortunately, good dosing guidelines for most drugs don't exist.

Children's doses are often determined by old and obsolete formulas. These formulas derive the child's dose by comparing the child's age or weight to an adult's. The "correct" dose is determined by multiplying this ratio by the adult dose. It doesn't take a genius to see that this is a less than perfect system.

A child's body is unique. You can't estimate your child's correct medication dose because he weighs half of what you do or because she is nearly a teenager. But we often do that and, worse yet, OTC manufacturers do it, too. (A notable exception is children's aspirin. The dosage guidelines on the side of the "baby" aspirin bottle were carefully considered. These are more precise than most other OTC products.)

What makes kids so different from adults?

To begin with the obvious, children have smaller bodies. A small error in dosing is seldom a problem for adults, but with children a ''small'' error is proportionately larger.

However, the problem is more complicated than just a difference in body size. A child's organ systems aren't fully matured. These organs may be the target for drug therapy, or they may be required to detoxify or eliminate the drugs once they've done their job.

Children usually have less efficient kidney and liver function, less water and proportionately more fat in their bodies, and less blood flow through critical organs than adults. All of these cause children to react to drugs and doses differently from the way adults do.

So how do you determine a proper dose of nonprescription medication for your child?

I wish I could tell you.

Unfortunately, little research has been done to determine children's doses for over-the-counter medications. Your only guide is to rely on the recommendations on the product label, as imperfect as they may be.

But there are still two things you can do.

The first is to watch your child closely for side effects of medication. This would be a lot easier if OTC manufacturers would list common side effects on the product's label. Unfortunately, they seldom do.

You should never give your child medication without knowing what side effects to expect. Throughout this book I have tried to indicate these, but no book can cover every side effect of every drug. However, you can get that information from the pharmacist who sells you the product.

Be sure to get this information *whenever* you buy an over-the-counter product. If your child experiences any side effect, stop giving the medication and get in touch with your pharmacist or doctor for further instructions.

The other thing you can do is to be sure you give the dose you think you're giving.

If you are to give a teaspoonful of medication to your child, be sure that that is just what you give. Pharmaceutical companies consider a teaspoonful to be 5.0 milliliters (ml.), no more and no less. Unfortunately, household teaspoons may measure between 3.5 and 8 milliliters. If you use these spoons, you would be giving your child anywhere from 70 percent to 160 percent of the correct dose. Therefore, you could end up either undertreating or overtreating your child.

Your best solution to this problem is to buy a specially designed medication measuring spoon from your local drugstore. These come in various shapes and sizes, and your pharmacist should be able to help you select the best one for your purpose.

Diaper Rash

No discussion of children's maladies would be complete without including diaper rash.

Diaper rash, or diaper dermatitis, is an acute skin rash in the diaper area that is characterized by intense inflammation and is often painful. Its exact cause has never been determined, but now we know some things that don't cause it.

It isn't caused by ammonia or urine, foods or food additives, or laundry detergents, although these can worsen a rash that is already there.

While we haven't been able to identify a specific cause, we do know that some factors make it worse. For instance, a rough diaper that constantly rubs against a baby's soft bottom makes the skin even more sensitive. Letting a baby sit in a wet or dirty diaper also irritates the skin and increases the chances of either developing a problem or making a preexisting rash worse.

Diaper rash pops up when a combination of factors is present. It may be that there is no single cause, that our children are victimized when we parents don't pay enough attention to prevention.

The best diaper rash prevention is plain common sense. Change your child's diaper whenever it's wet, and attach the new diaper loosely to prevent friction. Infants should also be changed at least one time during the night. Clean the child's bottom with soap and water after each changing, being sure to get into all the little cracks, crevices, and skin folds. And never use the dry part of a wet diaper to clean feces off the skin. This grinds bacteria into sensitive areas and can start a nasty rash.

One of the banes of baby's bottoms is plastic pants or liners over disposable diapers. These baby bloomers trap moisture inside the diaper and damage the skin. Exposure to excessive moisture damages skin and makes it easier for a rash to start. Plastic pants may be necessary at times, but limit your child's wearing time and never use them at night.

Diapers from a laundry service seem to cause fewer cases of diaper rash than do home laundered diapers. One reason is that the service diapers are almost sterile when they are delivered to your home, so there are no residual bacteria or yeasts on them. The commercial services also do a better job of rinsing irritating detergents off the diaper than you can in your washing machine at home.

But no matter what you do, your baby will probably develop diaper rash at some time. And the pharmaceutical industry will be right there to sell you something to slap on it.

The Treatment of Diaper Rash

Nondrug treatments are primarily aimed at aeration—in other words, getting as much drying air on the baby's behind as possible. This includes avoiding plastic pants and liners, changing diapers as soon as the baby wets or poops, and letting the baby take naps without any diaper on. (What a mess!)

Most parents quickly tire of this routine and skip directly to one of the following drug treatments.

Powders—For Moisture Absorption

We learned with our eldest that cornstarch seemed to work pretty well for diaper rash. Powders absorb water and help keep a mild rash dry. Her diaper rashes appeared to heal a little faster when we kept her well-powdered.

It wasn't until later that we learned that we were taking unnecessary risks. Cornstarch can be food for bacteria, which gobble it up and become healthier and stronger. This isn't what we had in mind.

Rather than cornstarch, you might consider using talc. But it has its problems, too. Kids can inhale the powder and develop lung problems. If you use commercial baby powders, do your best to control the amount of powder that gets into the air and never let the baby play with the powder bottle.

Barriers—Primarily for Protection of Healthy Skin

Zinc oxide ointment and plain petrolatum (Vaseline) are among the most effective and least expensive barrier products available. The barrier products are protectants, they keep urine, feces, detergents, and other irritants from coming in contact with the baby's skin.

They also have an important disadvantage. They trap moisture inside the skin, and moisture is the number one enemy in diaper rash.

Barriers seem to work best if they are used when the skin is relatively normal. They can be used in the early stages of diaper rash to prevent new outbreaks or applied when the rash is about to heal.

Some products contain extra ingredients that either provide no additional benefit or cause problems. For instance, there is no proof that vitamins A and D improve healing time, and there are indications that boric acid may be absorbed through the baby's skin and cause toxicity.

Anti-Inflammatory Treatment—Risk of Worse to Come

You may be tempted to use the anti-inflammatory drug hydrocortisone. Don't do it.

Hydrocortisone may take down your baby's inflammation quickly, but you also run the risk of making the problem worse in the long run. We now know that 85 percent of diaper rashes are contaminated with the yeast *Candida albicans,* the same organism that causes vaginal yeast infections in adult women. Hydrocortisone can limit the body's ability to fight off this yeast, making the diaper rash worsen after a temporary improvement.

Anti-Yeast Cream and Powder—Effective Treatment Agents

If yeast is such a big problem in diaper rash, wouldn't it be nice if we had something that could kill the microorganisms? Fortunately, we do.

Miconazole, the same drug that we use to treat athlete's foot, is an effective yeast killer. After the cornstarch debacle with our first child, we learned about the use of miconazole (brand name Micatin). We saw that diaper rashes didn't get as bad if they were treated early with miconazole and that they improved faster than with other products.

Micatin comes in various forms, but the two most useful ones for this application are the cream and the powder. You can use the cream for active cases of diaper rash, and the powder makes a decent anti-yeast dusting powder.

Miconazole seldom causes side effects. If you notice that it is causing irritation or appears to burn the baby at the site of application, wash it off thoroughly and discontinue use.

The Pharmacist's Prescription for Diaper Rash

Change your baby's diaper as soon as it gets wet or dirty.

Change your baby's diaper at least once during the night.

Attach the new diaper loosely to allow as much air to circulate as possible.

Use plastic pants only when absolutely necessary, and never at night or during naps.

If you launder your own diapers, make sure they are rinsed thoroughly. Put them through an extra rinse cycle.

Apply miconazole cream to diaper rash at every diaper change.

See the Doctor if . . .
- Your child's rash only occurs in patches.
- Your child's diaper rash lasts more than seventy-two hours after you start treatment.
- Your child has bumps or blisters on its bottom.
- Your child has open sores or oozes fluid.
- Your child has diarrhea.

Products Recommended for Diaper Rash

Baby Magic Lotion	Micatin Powder
Baby Magic Powder	Rexall Baby Powder
Diaparene Medicated Cream	Talc
Johnson's Baby Powder	Vaseline Pure Petroleum Jelly
Micatin Cream	Zincofax Cream

Or the generic equivalent of any of the above

Products Not Recommended for Home Medication of Diaper Rash

A and D Ointment (A)
Ammens Medicated Powder (D)
Borofax Ointment (D)
Desitin Ointment (I)
Diaparene Baby Powder (D)
Hydrocortisone cream or lotion (E)
Johnson and Johnson Medicated Powder (I)
Mexsana Medicated Powder (D)
Or the generic equivalent of any of the above

The products listed in the "Not Recommended" tables are not recommended by me for one or more of the following reasons: (A) One or more ingredients have been reported to be ineffective or only slightly effective for the product's intended purpose; (B) a more effective product is available; (C) the product advertising or description is likely to heighten consumer expectation beyond actual effectiveness; (D) the product has the potential to cause side effects in the average consumer that are more serious than those generally associated with OTC drugs; (E) the product has the potential to cause serious side effects in persons with specific diseases or disorders; (F) another product is available that is capable of producing the same or nearly the same therapeutic effect without the same risk of side effects; (G) persistent use of the product may cause physical dependency that alters an otherwise normal body function; (H) the product's formulation may reduce the effectiveness of one of its ingredients; (I) this is a multiple-ingredient product that may have no therapeutic advantage over simpler or single-ingredient products; (J) one or more of the product's ingredients may be useful for only a short period during the total duration of the illness; (K) the product cannot easily be administered at a dosage level within generally recommended boundaries of optimal therapeutic effect; (L) this is a condition-specific product that is appropriate for use only after a health professional has helped the patient establish a diagnosis.

Reye's Syndrome

Reye's (pronounced RIZE) syndrome is a rare brain disease that occurs most often in children under age sixteen who are recovering from viral influenza or chicken pox. Most cases occur during flu epidemics. Between 600 and 1200 cases occur each year and about one-fourth of these children die. Most of the survivors suffer permanent brain damage.

Since the early 1970s growing evidence has indicated a link between Reye's syndrome and the use of aspirin in children. The U.S. Public Health Service now advises parents not to give aspirin in any form to children who have the flu or chicken pox. Acetaminophen is a suitable alternative for these kids.

Does this mean that aspirin causes Reye's syndrome?

No, the cause is still not known. But we can't ignore the relationship between Reye's and aspirin use. However, avoidance of aspirin is no guarantee that an individual will not contact Reye's.

Hopefully, children's aspirin abstinence will decrease the number of cases per year.

Every parent should be aware of the possibility of Reye's because of its devastating effects. The early symptoms of Reye's are:

- Aggressive or assaultive behavior
- Lack of energy
- Persistent vomiting
- Unconsciousness
- Unexplained confusion

If your child should suddenly experience any of these symptoms, contact your doctor immediately. *Reye's syndrome is an emergency condition.* Early treatment can make the difference between life and death.

Poisoning

The National Clearinghouse for Poison Control Centers estimates that two-thirds of all accidental poison ingestions occur in children *under five years of age.*

This year more than 125,000 emergency calls will be made to poison control centers because of accidental poisonings in this age group. Worse yet, epidemiologists estimate that only one poisoning in ten is reported to a poison center.

Most of these incidents happen because an adult has been careless. Adults have to take responsibility for childhood poisonings. Almost 90 percent of all child poisonings occur when an adult is present.

We have to do better.

Poison Prevention

Common sense is the key to preventing poisoning. The tables below give some specific tips for prevention as well as a home checklist for identifying hazardous situations and locations in your home.

Poison Prevention Guidelines

Any product other than food may be a potential poison.

Keep all household products and medicines out of reach of children, preferably in child-resistant containers and locked in cabinets when not in use.

Store internal medication separately from household products.

Keep household products and medications in their original containers.

Read the label of all medications and household products before using them.

Always refer to medicines as "medicine." Never tell a child that medicine is candy.

Clean out the medicine cabinet periodically. Throw away expired drugs as well as those that you no longer use.

Do not carry medicine in your purse unless absolutely necessary.

Avoid taking medication in front of children.

Never take another person's medication.

Know the names of all the plants growing in and around your home.

Keep all medications in child-resistant containers.

Do not eat foods that look or smell unusual.

Never leave a poison within a child's reach, even for only a few seconds.

Mark potential poisons so your child can recognize them as hazardous.

Dispose of products that have lost their labels.

Use cleaning fluids and aerosols only in well-ventilated areas.

Do not spray pesticides or herbicides on windy days.

Never place rat, mouse, or insect poisons or traps where children can reach them.

Never "spike" or "bait" food with insecticides or pesticides.

Any drug, chemical, cleanser, disinfectant, plant, detergent, or other substance in your home is a potential child-killer. Poison prevention is a full-time job, a job that has no short cuts or holidays. And it is the responsibility of everyone in the home.

Children can get into places where they don't belong with lightning speed. You can't rely on seeing them or hearing them get into cabinets or drawers. By the time you find that your child has gotten into something he or she shouldn't have, it may be too late. The best attitude is to assume that children will get into toxins unless you take steps in advance to prevent it.

Fortunately, help is close at hand.

One of the best things you can do is to make your kitchen and storage cabinets and drawers child-resistant. Most pharmacies and hardware stores sell child-resistant latches that are hard for children under five to open. Some hardware stores also sell similar latches for your medicine chest, the most dangerous cubic foot in your house.

If you apply child-resistant latches throughout your home, you're off to a good start, but there's much more that needs to be done.

Inspect your house. But don't do it as an adult. Look at your house as if you were a child. What areas would interest you? What about the perfumes and colognes Mom keeps on her dresser? They are potential poisons. What about the can of gasoline Dad keeps in the garage for the lawnmower? That's even more dangerous than the perfume.

Look at every room. Do you know the names of all the plants in your home? Do you know which are toxic and which

A Home Checklist for Preventing Poisoning*

Kitchen:

No household products are kept under the sink.

No medications are left out on the counters.

All cleansers are out of reach.

All medications and cleaning products are kept in proper containers.

Poison control center phone number is posted by each telephone.

Bathroom:

Medicine chest is cleaned regularly.

Only currently used medications are kept.

Old medications are properly disposed of by flushing down the toilet.

All medications have child-resistant caps.

There is a child-resistant latch on the medicine cabinet.

A bottle of syrup of ipecac is kept in a safe place (see page 357).

Bedrooms and Living Room:

No medications are left out on the dresser, chest, or night stand.

All perfumes, colognes, and cosmetics are out of reach.

No flaking paint chips are in evidence on windowsills, woodwork, crib, or playpen.

All plants are identified, and dangerous plants are placed out of reach.

Laundry:

Soaps, detergents, and bleaches are out of reach.

All empty containers are washed out with water before disposal.

Garage and Basement Storage:

Following products are out of reach and preferably locked in cabinets:

Antifreeze	Insecticides	Paint thinner
Caulk	Kerosene	Soldering
Drain cleaners	Paint	compound
Gasoline	Paint stripper	"Super" glue
Herbicides		

*You may want to photocopy this list and check each item off on the photocopy as you make sure that you have followed the advice given here.

aren't? Do you know that a child can suffocate from biting into a leaf of a dumb cane (diffenbachia) plant?

If your child is at the crawling stage, he will be particularly interested in the lowlands. Do you keep detergents, solvents, insecticides, or cleansers on low shelves in the garage, kitchen, or laundry room?

What about grandparents? The same rules apply there. Every year thousands of kids get poisoned at Grandma's house. Why? Because grandparents forget about the things their kids used to get into.

The rules for poison prevention don't apply only to those households with small children—they apply to every home. Even if you don't have children, children still come into your house. You may be responsible for poisoning a niece or nephew or a neighbor's or a friend's child. And if you're too self-centered to be concerned with someone else's child, think about your legal liability.

Child-resistant containers became mandatory for most prescription and nonprescription drugs in 1973. Despite their inconvenience, these special caps have drastically decreased the number of children's poisonings involving medication. But they don't work unless you use them.

There are legitimate reasons for requesting that the pharmacist not put child-resistant caps on your medicine bottles. Arthritics, for instance, can have a difficult time getting these lids off their bottles. But many people who request easy-opening caps do so only for their own convenience. That defeats the purpose of the legislation.

Small children often mistake medicines for candy. They are attracted to a medicine bottle like a magnet. Anything we can do to make it more difficult for a child to get into medication saves lives. Child-resistant containers are life savers.

Who needs to use child-resistant containers? Obviously, parents of small children. But who else?

Grandparents, particularly grandmothers. Why is it so important for Grandma to use them? Because Grandma comes visiting with her medicines in her purse, that treasure trove of wondrous and mysterious things, which kids love to explore. When Grandma comes for an afternoon visit she may bring a toy, perhaps some candy. She also brings her hormones, blood pressure medication, and heart pills.

Do you carry "purse poisons" with you? Chances are that you do. A survey of 300 women accompanying children to a pediatric clinic showed that 191, or *over 60 percent*, carried at least one purse poison. Most of these women had never considered their purses to be a potential source of danger.

Look through your purse and take out any hazardous materials that you don't absolutely have to carry with you.

Now, what about this nonsense that only a child can open a child-resistant container?

You've heard the stories. "I can't get my medicine bottles open, so I give them to my eight-year-old. He doesn't have any trouble at all."

Of course not, they aren't intended for him.

First of all, I've encountered few adults who couldn't open one of these things if they took the time to read and follow the directions on the cap. Most people who have trouble with these containers don't pay attention to what they're doing. Don't expect to get too much sympathy from pharmacists. We open hundreds of them each day.

Second, these caps are "child-*resistant*," not "child-*proof*." They are only intended to slow the kids down, not to make the containers impenetrable.

Child-resistant containers are designed for children under five, the group at highest risk of poisoning. Before these containers are permitted to be sold on the market, their manufacturers have to prove that 80 percent of children less than five years of age cannot open them in less than five minutes. They also have to prove that more than 80 percent of adults can open them in that same time period.

My nine-year-old doesn't have any problem with these caps, either. But my six- and four-year-olds can't get them off, and they're the ones I'm most concerned about, since they are too young to understand verbal warnings.

What Do You Do If a Poisoning Occurs?

The best advice I can give you is to assume that you will have a poisoning in your house—and pray that it doesn't happen.

You can't handle a poison situation if you aren't prepared.

The two most important things for you to do ahead of time are to write the name and telephone number of your regional poison control center next to the phone. You can find this information on the inside front cover of your telephone directory.

The second thing is to buy a bottle of syrup of ipecac. Ipecac is an emetic; it makes the victim vomit. Emetics are effective first aid measures for most poisons, but they can make others worse. How do you know which case you're dealing with? *Call your doctor or poison control center before you do anything.*

The poison control center will want some information from you. Be prepared to tell them the time the poisoning occurred, what and how much was taken, and how the victim feels. At this point they'll make some recommendations to you. That's where the ipecac comes in. If the staff at the poison center feels that you should get the victim to vomit, tell them that you have some ipecac and ask for directions. They'll tell you how much to use and what to expect.

Never make a poison victim vomit unless a health professional advises you to do so.

What if you can't tell if your child has actually swallowed something? Call the poison center and explain the situation. They'll advise you on a proper course of action.

When a Poisoning Occurs

Keep the victim quiet.

Calmly determine what and how much was taken.

Call your doctor or your local poison control center, giving them the information you have.

If instructed to go to the hospital or doctor's office, take the poison container along with any vomited material.

Bring a container in case the victim vomits on the way to the hospital.

Do not induce vomiting or start any treatment unless advised to do so by a doctor or poison control center.

Some Tip-offs That Your Child Has Been Poisoned

What if you don't know that your child has gotten into something. How can you tell if he or she has been poisoned? The list below can give you some help. If your child shows any of the indicated symptoms of poisoning, *call your doctor or poison center immediately.*

Alertness is the key. If you are both attentive to the toxic substances in your home—know what they are and where they are properly stored—*and* to your child's behavior, you stand the best chance of recognizing that a poisoning may have occurred. Recognize that possibility when you see that

- Containers of potential poisons have been removed, opened, or spilled.
- Your child exhibits:
  Dizziness or unusual drowsiness
  Rapid or slow breathing
  Stains or burns on clothes, skin, or around the mouth
  Stomach pain
  Sudden change in behavior or consciousness
  Unusual odor on the breath, clothes, or skin
  Vomiting

Only one, or even none, of the above may be present.

Index

For easier reference, product brand names have been set in boldface type.